1974

be kept

LASERS

LASERS

O. S. Heavens

CHARLES SCRIBNER'S SONS
NEW YORK

First published in 1971 by
Gerald Duckworth & Company Limited
3 Henrietta Street, London W.C.2

© *1971 O. S. Heavens*

1 3 5 7 9 11 13 15 17 19 I/C 20 18 16 14 12 10 8 6 4 2

Printed in Great Britain
Library of Congress Catalog Card Number 73-2053
SBN 684-13399-7

Contents

List of Colour Plates

Preface

In the decade since the first laser was operated, the impact of this remarkable device has been felt not only in the laboratories of the physicists but in an ever widening field. The main developments which led to our understanding of light, and of optical phenomena, occurred a long time ago. The more glamorous fields of nuclear and particle physics had tended to displace the study of optics, which had reached the stage of consolidation and development of the basic underlying ideas. It seemed unlikely that any dramatic changes would occur and in some senses the field became an unfashionable one. The arrival of the laser marked a come-back, the extent of which can be judged from the enormous effort which was devoted to its study. Over five thousand papers appeared in the learned journals within the first ten years after discovery. Expenditure on development of the device approached five hundred million pounds within that time. The laser field became, within a very short time, one in which any kind of prediction was hazardous, so rapid and unexpected were many of its developments. A wide range of experiments and devices became possible over-night, many of them so far beyond the possibilities existing in the pre-laser era that they had never even been considered. The importance of the laser as a scientific development was signalled, in 1969, by the award of a Nobel Prize to the three pioneers— C. H. Townes in the U.S.A. and A. M. Prokhorov and N. Basov, in the U.S.S.R.—showing the high regard of the

Preface

world's scientific fraternity for this work.

In the past few years many books on lasers and laser devices have appeared. With one or two exceptions they have been aimed at the trained scientist or engineer and have presupposed a formal training in one or other of these disciplines, together with a sound mathematical background. This book is intended for the reader without such training and background, to enable him to learn, in general terms, how lasers work, how they are likely to develop, what they can do and what impact they are likely to have in the future. I hope that the brief introductory chapters on the nature of light will, despite their brevity, provide a suitable frame of reference for the subsequent discussion. The aim throughout is to give as far as possible a complete account in elementary terms, rather than to restrict to oversimplified models or handwaving explanations. The selection of topics is basic in the hope that, by avoiding the temptation to aim at presenting a comprehensive picture, the result will be sufficiently concise to serve the reader with a general interest. A bibliography of more advanced works is given at the end of the book.

It is a pleasure to thank Audrey Price for producing, often from the roughest of sketches, the line drawings and David Crowther and Matthew Hill for producing the colour plates.

O. S. Heavens.
September, 1970.

CHAPTER ONE

Introduction

In 1960, in the laboratories of the Hughes Aircraft Co., in California, an experiment was done with results which have made an enormous impact on the scientific world. The experiment was remarkably simple in concept. A synthetic ruby crystal, 2 cm long and 9 mm in diameter was inserted inside a helical flash tube, similar to those used for flash photography as shown in Fig. 1.1. The ends of the ruby rod had been carefully polished so they were exactly square to the axis and were coated with silver. When a flash was set off in the helical tube, a very brief pencil of deep red light emerged from the end of the ruby rod. This was the first successful demonstration of a laser—the first of what has proved to be an impressive series of devices with remarkable and striking properties and which have already transformed whole areas of science and technology.

The word "laser" is taken from the initials of the phrase describing the device—*l*ight *a*mplification by the *s*timulated *e*mission of *r*adiation. In the ensuing chapters we shall study the fascinating way in which these devices operate. We shall see that in some respects it is surprising that the laser did not arrive on the scene much earlier than 1960. At that date the underlying principles which account for the operation of the laser had been known and understood for no less than 43 years. When Einstein introduced the concept of stimulated emission in 1917, whereby a beam of light can induce atoms to give out similar radiation, this appeared to be of little importance other than to

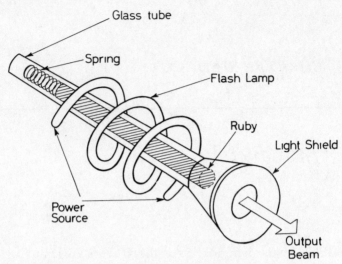

Fig. 1.1   Schematic of the first laser ever operated.

tidy up some discrepancies in theories extant at that time. Many years passed before the implications of Einstein's ideas on this subject were fully appreciated. With the wisdom of hindsight, we may say that some at least of our present lasers *could* have been built over forty years ago. The principles were known and the technology (which is in some cases rather simple) was already established. It seems possible, if not very likely, that the laser could have been discovered by accident and one may speculate happily on the influence which this would have had on the course of scientific research in the last few decades. We resist this temptation and turn our attention to the laser itself— how it functions and why it has made such an impact. Before discussing the "how", it will help if we examine in some detail the way in which light-producing devices work and discuss some of the features of beams of light and other kinds of radiation. Let us first, however, indicate the features of the laser which amply justify the intense interest and excitement which its arrival has heralded.

The laser is a device which produces an intense, highly directional beam of light of a very pure colour. The laser beam also possesses the property of coherence, which indicates a certain regularity of the waves in the beam.

Although the description in this form may not seem remarkable, the laser differs from any other kind of light source in all four characteristics mentioned above, and in ways which have quite dramatic impacts.

Consider for example the directional aspect. A typical laser beam may be only 1 mm diameter at the point where it leaves the laser and may spread to only about half a centimetre in diameter at a distance of 10 m (Fig. 1.2). In practically every other light source, light emerges in all directions, although not necessarily uniformly. The familiar filament lamp can be seen from all directions. The projector lamp succeeds in sending out more light in one direction than another, but this is achieved by suitable shaping of the filament. Each point on the filament radiates uniformly—it is just that we can see more emitting area from the front than from the side. By a suitable use of lenses or mirrors, we can obtain a directional beam of light from a filament lamp, as in a torch or searchlight. However, the source itself—the lamp, or carbon arc—sends its light in all directions. In contrast, the intense light from the laser emerges *only* in the fine pencil-like beam.

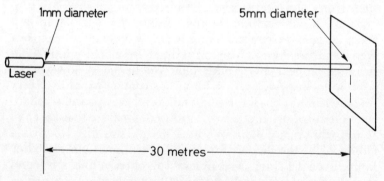

1mm diameter   5mm diameter

Laser

←————————30 metres————————→

Fig. 1.2   All the light from the laser emerges in a very narrow beam.

Because the laser gives out light into such a narrow beam, it appears as an extremely intense source. If we look at a 100-watt lamp filament at a distance of 1 ft (30 cm) the power entering the eye is less than a thousandth of a watt, because the light from the lamp streams out more or less uniformly in all directions. *If* we were to look directly along the beam from a laser (which we never do) then *all* the radiated power would enter the eye. Thus even a 1-watt laser would appear many thousand times more intense than the 100-watt ordinary lamp.

Extremely high intensity laser beams may be produced, either as continuous sources or in the form of flashes of very short duration. The most powerful pulsed laser flashes will vaporise any known material and have, for example, been used to drill holes in diamond, the hardest material known. An impressive continuous laser is that which uses a tube of carbon dioxide, nitrogen and helium. With this device—which produces an invisible, infra-red beam—holes may be drilled through firebricks within a matter of seconds.

No less remarkable than the high intensity capability of the laser is that of producing a beam of extremely pure colour. If the light from an ordinary filament lamp is examined in a spectroscope, as Newton first examined sunlight in the seventeenth century, a continuous colour range is seen, from violet through blue, green, yellow and orange, to red as in Plate 1*a*. The different colours are found to correspond to different wavelengths of the light, from about four hundred-thousandths of a centimetre for violet light to seven hundred-thousandths for red. In contrast, if we examine the light from a mercury lamp in a spectroscope, we see a small number of lines (Plate 1*b*) each of a well-defined colour. These are termed "monochromatic" and do indeed appear as very pure colours to the eye. If, however, we were to look very closely, with an instrument capable of very fine discrimination, we should find that these apparently sharp lines often consisted of a small group of separate lines, each of slightly different colour, or wavelength. Thus Fig. 1.3 gives a close look at the "monochromatic" green line from an iodine lamp. Even if a close inspection reveals only *one* line, it is found that the line is never perfectly sharp, but that it always spreads a little. A similar inspection of the light from a laser would reveal virtually no spreading at all—the light is vastly more monochromatic than that of any conventional line source. Fig. 1.4 gives an idea of the relative widths of lines from non-laser and from laser sources. The implications of this property of the laser are examined in Chapter 13 where it will be seen that the laser provides us with a powerful tool for precision measurement over long distances.

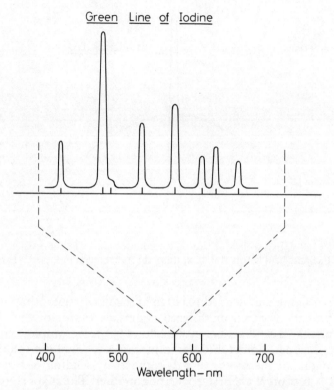

Fig. 1.3 Fine structure in the yellow line from an iodine spectrum. What appears at first sight to be a single yellow line is in fact a group of very fine components.

The fourth laser characteristic which distinguishes it from ordinary light sources is coherence. When one looks at the light from an ordinary source, the eye receives enormous numbers of waves, coming from myriads of different atoms in the source. Each of the atoms gives out a train of light waves at intervals but a strict state of non-co-operation exists among the atoms, which behave with a rugged individuality. Each sends out its light wave just when the atom thinks fit, with no reference to any of its neighbours. Thus although a single stone dropped into a pond gives a regular, well-defined pattern of waves, the effect of a continuous stream of stones falling in from a shute is one of chaos so far as wave regularity is concerned. From the briefest of

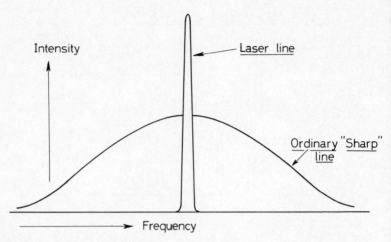

Fig. 1.4 Relative widths of laser and non-laser lines. (In some cases, the laser line may be a hundred million times sharper than an ordinary "sharp" line.)

intervals, one may see a tiny patch of regularity but for most of the time the waves from different atoms are thoroughly mixed up, giving us an "incoherent" beam of light. In complete contrast, the operation of the laser imposes a strict discipline on the behaviour of the atoms, which respond by sending out their light-waves precisely in step with one another. The chaos is gone and the resultant light-wave has a beautiful regularity, rising and falling in perfect sequence, for as long as the laser is working. In this respect the radiation from the laser shows a close resemblance to the waves which are used for radio transmission. Both are coherent. This may suggest that laser radiation could perhaps be used, in some circumstances, instead of radio waves and this is indeed the case. As we shall see in Chapter 13, laser waves possess truly enormous potential for just this purpose.

CHAPTER TWO

The nature of light

> My Design in this Book is not to explain the Properties of Light
> by Hypotheses, but to propose and prove them by Reason and
> Experiments. . . .   Isaac Newton, *Opticks*, 4th ed., 1730.

In Newton's famous treatise, a whole range of experiments are
described which show clearly many of the rules of behaviour
followed by beams of light. They illustrate the way in which
light is reflected at a mirror, refracted, as at a glass or water
surface, and dispersed, or split up into its constituent colours.
The experiments showed how a light beam does not cast a
perfectly sharp shadow, even if a minute source is used, but
spreads slightly into the shadow, often with alternations of light
and dark—a phenomenon known as diffraction. They showed,
too, that beams of light could interact with one another to produce light and dark, as in the celebrated Newton's Rings
experiment, illustrated in Plate 2. Newton observed that ring
patterns of different sizes formed, depending on the colour of
light used, and he discovered the law governing the diameters
of the rings—that the squares of the diameters are in the ratio
$1 : 2 : 3 : 4 : \ldots$ This phenomenon, of interference, is one which
in many ways gives one of the most dramatic of illustrations of
the wave property of light. Not only do patterns of interference
fringes *look* like waves, but their explanation can be very simply
given in terms of waves. Direct analogies exist between the
behaviour of waves on water and waves of light. Strangely
enough (as it now seems) Newton's descriptions of the phenomena which he investigated so completely experimentally were
made not in terms of waves but of corpuscles, or light "particles". The fact that part of a light beam was reflected at a glass

7

surface and part transmitted was ascribed to "fits of easy reflexion" and "fits of easy transmission". ("And hence Light is in Fits of easy Reflexion and easy Transmission, before its Incidence on transparent Bodies. And probably it is put into such fits at its first emission from luminous Bodies, and continues in them during all its progress.") At a later stage, Huyghens proposed an explanation of the behaviour of light in terms of waves. A crucial result enabling a choice between the alternative models of waves and particles emerged when the velocity of light in, e.g., glass compared with that in a vacuum was considered. The fact that light bent towards the normal to a surface on entering glass from air (or vacuum) indicated, on a wave picture, that it travelled more slowly in glass than in air. On the particle picture, it had to be assumed, to account for the observed bending, that light travelled *faster* in glass. ("If light be swifter in bodies than in vacuo, in the proportion of the sines which measure the refraction of the bodies, the forces of the bodies to reflect and refract light are very nearly proportional to the densities of the bodies; except that unctuous and sulphureous bodies refract more than others of the same density"!) When it was shown that light indeed travels more *slowly* in "bodies" than in vacuo, the argument appeared to be settled and the wave theory became the "correct" description. Further powerful and elegant confirmation of wave ideas came when Maxwell, in 1860, gave his electromagnetic theory of light, which showed that, starting with the basic known laws of electricity and magnetism, one was led inexorably to the idea that waves of electrical/magnetic effects would travel at precisely the speed at which light was observed to go and would show all the properties which Newton had demonstrated—refraction, reflection, diffraction, interference, etc. So complete and satisfactory did electromagnetic theory appear that it must have come as a shock when experimental results began to turn up which stubbornly refused to fit a picture which accounted for so many observations so successfully. Before the present century was very old, it had begun to dawn that in some ways beams of light behaved very much as though they consisted of streams of particles, or "quanta". The details of these experiments need not concern us. Nor need we delve into the problems of visualisation which are encountered in describing the "true" nature of light. We need not expect always to see the same aspect of behaviour of the systems which we observe—much will depend on what we are doing with them—on the *kind* of way we are looking at them. If we put the mirrors or slits in the way of a beam in the way which shows up interference fringes, we shall be conscious of the wave properties of light. If we put an electron in the way, it is kicked out of the way by the light as though hit by a particle. In one experiment we "see" the wave aspect and in the other the quantum aspect. We never see both at the same time.

One of the neatest direct experiments showing the wave character of light is Wiener's. This makes use of the fact that if two similar waves travel along the same line in opposite directions, we get a fixed, "standing-wave" pattern, as shown in Fig. 2.1. In this case the waves are sent along a string and the

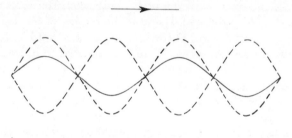

Fig. 2.1 Standing waves. The resultant wave oscillates between the dotted extremes, without moving sideways.

result is that at some places the string is still whilst at others, midway between the stationary points, it swings madly from side to side. This suggests that if we do this with two light beams, we should get light and dark regions. The experiment is difficult because the bright parts are rather close together but the effect was successfully demonstrated. Wiener used a mirror so that the light reflected from it formed the reversed beam. The beams traversed a photographic emulsion and so took their own photograph, with the result as shown in Fig. 2.2.

Satisfying though it is to account for the behaviour of light in terms of waves, one must face the question "waves of *what*?" In the early days of the wave theory, space was imagined to be

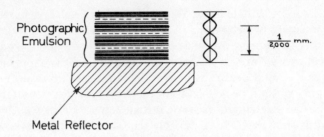

Fig. 2.2   Schematic of standing light waves in Wiener's experiment. The light and dark bands form in the photographic emulsion.

filled with an elastic fluid which served to transmit the waves from place to place. This idea ran into difficulties when attempts were made to characterise the "fluid" which would have had to behave enormously differently from any known material. When Maxwell's theory was developed, it was seen that the waves associated with light could simply be waves of electric and magnetic disturbances. Disturbances of this kind could be established in a vacuum, so there was no need to insist on the idea of a "fluid" (which would have to be present in vacuum as well as elsewhere) to enable the waves to be transmitted.

Maxwell's picture, then, of a light wave—one of a single colour—is that of a wave of electric and magnetic fields, streaming into space at a velocity of 300,000 km/sec, or 186,000 miles/sec. If we were able to "freeze" the wave in an instant of time it would look like that in Fig. 2.3. The distance between successive maxima of the wave is termed the wavelength (λ).

Alternatively, we may imagine ourselves sitting in the path of the light beam with a device for measuring the electric (or magnetic) field. As time passed, we should observe the field varying rapidly in a wave-like fashion, so that a plot would appear as in Fig. 2.4. The number of waves passing each second is the frequency of the wave (v). If v waves go by in a second and each is of length λ, then the wave moves a distance $v \times \lambda$ in a second: in other words

velocity = frequency × wavelength.

Although we have been referring mostly to light, Maxwell's ideas on electromagnetic waves turn out to be applicable to a whole range of waves of which light forms a minute part. At one

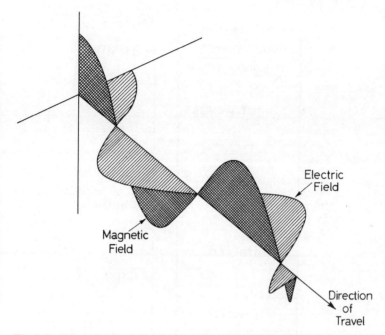

Fig. 2.3 "Snapshot" of electromagnetic wave in space. The wave moves along the "direction of travel" with a velocity of 300,000 km/sec.

end of the scale we have radio waves, with wavelengths from tens to hundreds of metres long; at the other end is the very short wavelength radiation which streams in from outer space. In between the extremes we have, in order of increasing wavelength, X-rays, ultra-violet, visible and infra-red regions of the spectrum. Fig. 2.5 shows the spectrum of electromagnetic waves with which we are familiar, with the names allotted to the

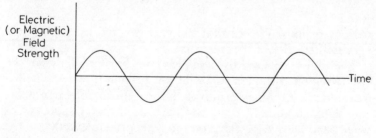

Fig. 2.4 Variation of amplitude of wave at a given point as time passes.

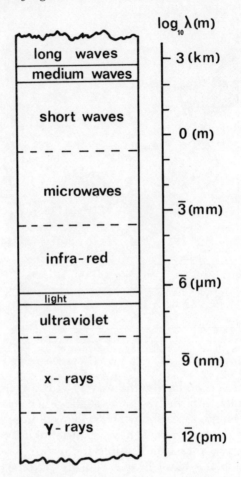

Fig. 2.5   The Electromagnetic Spectrum.

various regions. We see that the part covered by "light" is a
very limited slice of the spectrum.

The region covered by lasers is somewhat broader than the
visible region, although still small. At present it extends from a
wavelength of about $\frac{1}{4000}$ mm, in the near ultra-violet part of the
spectrum, to about 1 mm, approaching the very short radio-
wave part. Devices working on the same principle as that of the
laser have been made to work at longer wavelengths—to about

one centimetre. As this falls in what is termed the microwave region, these devices are referred to as masers.

To summarise our description, then, of light and associated radiation, we can describe this as a wave-like disturbance, which travels through space at a speed of 300,000 km/sec. The waves are of electric and magnetic effects which oscillate at a rate which is connected with the wavelength (or in the visible region the colour) of the radiation. In the same way that waves on water may interfere with one another, or may spread round obstacles, so do light waves. We note that ultra-violet waves, light-waves and radio-waves are all fundamentally similar, differing only in respect of wavelength. We shall see that there are in fact some differences between, say, radio-waves and light-waves from ordinary light sources—differences other than that of wavelength. Before we examine this feature, we must first take a look at the sources themselves. We have so far confined our discussion to the behaviour of radiation after it has left the source. Since the laser is remarkable as a light source, we must look in detail on what goes on in the ordinary sources of light around us.

CHAPTER THREE

Sources of light

The earliest source of light of which man will have been conscious is the sun, which appears luminous to us simply by virtue of the fact that it is very hot. We make use of many similar sources, such as the ordinary electric lamp, with a heated filament as the emitter. Such sources appear white to us although we are aware of the fact that things at lower temperatures (such as an electric fire bar) appear red. If we examine sunlight, or the light from a "white" light filament source, with a spectroscope, we see a complete spectrum of colours ranging from red through orange, yellow, green and blue, to violet. In fact we are able to detect radiation outside this band of colours. We detect heating in the region beyond the red, where no visible effect is observed.

If we equip ourselves with instruments for measuring radiation at all wavelengths, we find that hot bodies give out a wide range of wavelengths, extending far outside the small visible range, and we find, moreover, that the intensities at different wavelengths depend only on the temperature of the source. Fig. 3.1 shows how the intensity emitted depends on wavelength for three different temperatures and we see from these curves why the colour of a hot source changes as the temperature is raised. The lowest curve, which corresponds roughly to the temperature of an electric fire bar, shows that more red light is emitted than other colours. At the intermediate temperature indicated, a different distribution of colours emerges and the eye registers this as white. At a higher temperature still, the maximum of the curve shifts further to shorter wavelengths, so that the light emitted appears bluish—as is seen in the electric arc used for welding.

Sources of this kind are called thermal sources and the graphs in Fig. 3.1 are termed Planck curves, after Max Planck,

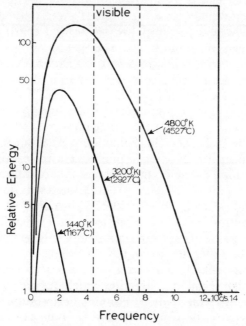

Fig. 3.1 Energy of radiation at different wavelengths for a thermal source (Planck curves).

who first derived the form of the curves. We shall in due course return to a discussion of the light emitted by the sun, for which the emission spectrum follows a Planck curve corresponding to a temperature of 6,000°C. (In fact, the curve is a Planck curve only provided we do not look too closely at it: the slight differences—sharp dark lines crossing the spectrum—have an important bearing on the question of what happens to light as it goes through matter.) For the moment, let us note that thermal sources give out a continuous spectrum of radiation, with a very wide range of wavelengths present, which we observe through our very limited visual window.

If we turn our spectroscope on to the familiar sodium street lamp, we get a very different result. From the visual effect produced we should certainly expect to see a preponderance of yellow in the spectrum. In fact we see just yellow, and nothing else. At first sight, we simply see one sharp yellow line: a really close look, provided the instrument is sensitive enough, reveals two lines extremely close together. If we examine instead the light from a helium lamp, we see several sharp lines—red, yellow, green, blue and violet. The spectra of light from these sources are shown in Plates 3 and 4. Examination of the light from a neon sign reveals a crowd of lines at the red end of the spectrum and practically nothing elsewhere. Since a discharge in a given gas or vapour always produces lines in the same parts of the spectrum, it is clear that these lines are a characteristic of the atom itself. In fact, this behaviour reveals a somewhat unexpected property of atoms—unexpected if we think of them simply as small particles, like minute billiard balls.

When we pass an electric current through sodium or mercury vapour, the electrons which make up the current try to stream down the tube from one electrode to the other. On the way however, they make an enormous number of collisions with the gas atoms in the tube. In some of these collisions, the electrons and atoms behave like billiard balls—the electrons bounce off the atoms, which recoil in a direction which depends on the direction of the electron at the collision. The recoiling atom is unchanged as a result of the collision. In some cases, however, a different behaviour is observed. If the incoming electron has sufficient energy, the state of the atom may be changed by the collision. The atom consists of a positively charged nucleus with a distribution of electrons around it. In its normal state, the surrounding electrons form a certain well-defined pattern round the nucleus, rather like a system of planets round the sun. The result of the collision with an incoming electron may be that the distribution of electrons round the atom changes and the atom is then said to be in an *excited state*. In this state, the atom possesses more energy than in the normal ("ground") state and is unstable. After a very short time (of the order of a hundred-millionth of a second) the atom spontaneously changes back to the normal state. In order that this shall happen, the excess energy which the atom had in the excited state must be dissipated and this is done by the emission of radiation. This may be visible light or radiation in other parts of the spectrum. Since the spectral lines emitted are characteristics of the emitting atom, the materials may be identified by the line emitted. In fact this form of analysis—spectrochemical analysis —provides us with an extremely powerful tool for studying the composition of matter. Thus in the manufacture of steel, it is essential to ensure that certain elements such as carbon are present in the right amounts and that other elements which have an adverse effect on the properties of the steel are absent. Spectrographic analysis forms a routine method of inspection in this situation.

There are other ways in which atoms may be excited and so produce emission spectra, other than by passing a current through the vapour of the material. If common salt is dropped through a hot flame, yellow emission occurs, similar to that from the sodium lamp. In this case, the energy needed for producing excited sodium atoms comes simply from collisions with the atoms in the flame which, because of the very high temperature of the flame, have very high velocities. They can, on collision with the sodium atoms from the salt, raise them to excited states in the same way that the electrons do in the discharge tube. Yet another way is by the use of light itself to produce excited atoms. We are familiar with the fluorescent paint materials commonly used in advertising. These paints contain small crystals with atoms capable of being raised to excited states by the absorption of the light falling on them. Sometimes the radiation absorbed is in the ultra-violet region of the spectrum. After absorbing the excited light, the atoms return to the normal state in two or more stages, in one or more of which the atom may give out visible light. This effect is seen in particularly beautiful form if materials such as starch, eggshell and most gemstones are exposed to a mercury lamp which is filtered to give *only* ultra-violet light. The eye sees no light actually falling on the crystals, but sees the fluorescence emitted as a mysterious, ghostly glow.

We shall return to a closer look at the way in which certain fluorescent materials behave, since these represent a large and important class of laser materials. Ruby is one of the most striking of these and the operation of the ruby laser depends directly on the fluorescent process outlined above. This is not the whole story, because the fluorescent light emitted by an ordinary piece of ruby streams out in all directions. We shall see later how we are able to arrange matters so that the majority of the light emitted streaks out in an intense, fine pencil. Before we do this, we must first look at the receiving end of the light from sources such as those described above.

CHAPTER FOUR

How things behave when exposed to light

We are familiar with a range of materials—air, glass, water— which appear to do practically nothing to a light beam which falls on them. The world seems almost the same through our bedroom window, whether or not this is open. We describe these materials as transparent, indicating that light which falls on them goes through "without let or hindrance". In fact we must realise that we can judge this only for the small range of wavelengths to which our eyes are sensitive. A perfectly transparent material would be one which allowed radiation of *all* wavelengths to pass freely through it. In fact the only material to which this definition applies is empty space (and there are even some reservations to this statement).

In general, materials are transparent to radiation in some part of the spectrum and absorbing in others. Although air appears quite transparent to us, it does not, in fact, allow ultra-violet radiation to pass freely through it—a fortunate feature for the inhabitants of the earth's surface, for whom undiluted sunlight would, because of its ultra-violet content, be harmful. Sometimes, materials which appear completely opaque to visible light are quite transparent in some other region. Ebonite—quite black and opaque to light even in very thin sheets—is transparent in the infra-red region of the spectrum, as are germanium and silicon. The latter materials, which form the basis of modern electronic technology, appear almost metallic to the eye, and let practically no visible light through, even in layers one hundredth of a millimetre thick; but they allow certain infra-red radiation through as freely as glass lets through visible light.

The extent to which materials are capable of transmitting light varies enormously, depending on the wavelength and on the nature of the material. If we confine our attention for the moment to visible light, we can make some rough generalisations. Metals are without exception almost completely opaque to visible radiation. A layer of silver only a ten-thousandth of a millimetre thick would be almost opaque—one would just see a very bright light through it. The so-called "one-way" mirrors, redolent of the gambling-house, consist of a metal film (usually silver) much thinner than this, Fig. 4.1. The name "one-way"

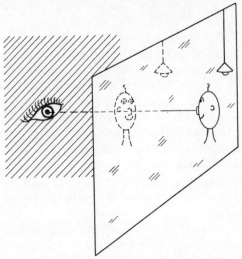

Fig. 4.1 The "one-way" mirror. The eye is in a darkened room. Very little light from this room gets through to the man in the brightly-lit room, who sees only the reflection of the room he is in. In the darkened room, there is hardly any light to *be* reflected. The watcher can therefore see the lighted room very clearly.

may suggest that light passes through more easily in one direction than the other. This is not in fact the case. If the observer sits on one side of such a mirror in a darkened room, he cannot be seen from the other—brightly lit—side. Most of the light which falls on the mirror is reflected. Sufficient gets through for the observer to see the lighted room—a very small fraction suffices for this. Although this small amount illuminates the observer, it is insufficient for him to become visible from the brightly-lit side, from which the wooer of the goddess of Chance will see only his own, brightly-lit and hopeful reflection in the mirror.

This digression serves to remind us of a further behaviour of materials to a light beam—the ability to reflect light. What, we ask, happens to light which fails to penetrate the material upon which it falls? In all cases, *some* of the light is reflected and in the case of metals, this may amount to a large fraction. Silver is the most popular material used for making mirrors because it reflects about 95% of visible light falling on it. Aluminium runs a close second, giving about 90% reflection. Although chromium plating is widely used for producing highly reflecting surfaces, it is a much poorer reflector than either silver or aluminium.

All the metals mentioned above reflect the colours making up visible light roughly equally. There are, however, metals which reflect some colours more strongly than others. Thus the ruddy hue of a copper surface arises simply because it reflects light at the red end of the visible spectrum much more strongly than the blue end. Gold, brass and bronze are other examples of metals which reflect different colours unequally.

But what happens to the light which is *not* reflected by a metal. We know that, if the metal layer is thin enough, some light can actually pass through it, but this is clearly not so for a thick slab. Some of the light energy falling on a metal is always absorbed. We can understand how this happens by noting (1) that metals are good conductors of electricity and (2) that light waves involve electric (and magnetic) fields. When a light wave tries to go through a piece of metal, the electric field of the light wave tries to set up electric currents in the metal. It can do this because metals contain electrons which are able to move around rather easily—they are not tied very tightly to the metal atoms as electrons are in other materials. However the metal atoms do get in the way of the currents of electrons set up by the light wave—the electrons keep colliding with the metal atoms and cause them to bounce around more than they normally do. This is another way of saying that the metal becomes heated. In fact, the energy of the metal simply re-appears as heat. For any ordinary intensities of light beams, the heating effects are very small. We shall see later (Chapter 13) that with the very intense beams obtainable from a laser, the heating effect can be very large—so much so that it is possible to vaporise the metal with a laser beam. Although metals form rather a special class of materials, the general property—that the light energy which is not reflected nor transmitted through the material causes heating—is one applying to many materials. When white light falls on blue paint, much of the blue part of the light is thrown back. The red, orange, yellow etc., part of the light striking the paint is absorbed and produces slight heating in the material.

We saw earlier—in discussing the way in which the sodium or mercury lamp worked—that we can describe what goes on in terms of the formation of excited atoms. We can still do this to account for the way in which light is absorbed by matter. The light energy taken up produces excited atoms (or groups of atoms). When the atoms fall back to their normal state, the excess energy goes into making all the atoms in the material vibrate a little faster—i.e. the temperature of the material is raised.

For substances which are highly transparent, the amount of light energy converted into heat is very small. Thus if we send a beam of white light on to a sheet of ordinary, clear glass, we find, on measuring the light passing through it, that this amounts to about 92% of the light striking the glass. This does not mean that the remaining 8% is absorbed, because some light is reflected, even by clear glass. The total amounts to about 8%, so the sum of the reflected and transmitted portions amounts almost exactly to the amount incident on the glass. Very little light is absorbed. If however we examine a piece of deep red glass we may well find that for red light the reflected and transmitted light practically equals the amount of incident red light, whereas for blue light we may have only 4% reflected and very little transmitted. Most of the energy of the incident blue light (or the blue part of an incident white light beam) is actually absorbed.

For the most part, the processes which we have been discussing so far in this chapter are those in which the effects produced on the light arise because of the properties of the atoms

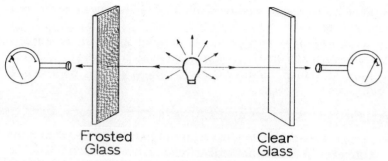

Fig. 4.2   Light transmitted by sheet of frosted glass. The detector is measuring the light going straight through.

making up the material in question. We can sum up the results by saying that

$$\text{Reflection} + \text{Transmission} + \text{Absorption} = 100\%$$

We have, however, ignored one other property possessed by some materials which concerns their ability to scatter light. Clear glass and frosted glass consist of exactly the same kinds of atoms and we should not expect frosted glass to absorb light appreciably. However we certainly cannot see things clearly through frosted glass. If we were to direct a narrow beam of light on to frosted glass and were to place (Fig. 4.2) a small detector behind the glass, we should record a very low transmission compared with that for clear glass. On the other hand if we were to measure (Fig. 4.3) the light reflected at the front surface

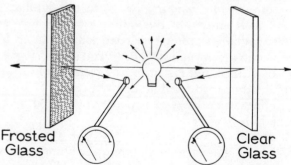

Fig. 4.3   Light reflected by sheet of frosted glass. Since the light neither goes straight through nor is reflected by the frosted glass, it seems that much of it must be lost. In fact it is scattered in all directions.

of the frosted glass, we should find that almost the same amount is reflected as in the case of clear glass. There is clearly a large balance of light energy not accounted for. This balance is *scattered*—it all comes out of the glass but is scattered in all directions. Thus to give a more complete story, we should formulate our balance sheet as

Reflected + Transmitted + Absorbed + Scattered = 100%

Highly scattering materials take light which is incident from a given direction and redistribute it over a wide range of directions—in complete contrast to the smooth glass or metal layer, which reflects in a specific direction. The latter process is termed specular reflection.

Sometimes, scattering in a material, such as a gem stone, arises from the presence of faults or imperfections in the material. In materials for use as lasers, the effects of scattering can appreciably reduce the efficiency of the laser. Great care is needed in the preparation of laser materials to ensure that scattering effects are reduced to a minimum.

There remains one other important way in which a beam of light may interact with matter. In this, the light energy is absorbed by atoms of the material and raises the atoms to excited states. In returning to the ground state, the atoms may emit some (or all) of the energy absorbed in the form of light of other colours, or wavelengths. Thus if we take a tube containing sodium vapour and expose it to a beam of ultra-violet radiation with a wavelength of 337 nm (which is invisible to the eye) we find that the sodium vapour glows with the familiar yellow colour such as is emitted by the sodium lamp. In this case, the ultra-violet radiation produces excited sodium atoms some of which return to the normal state in several stages (Fig. 4.4). In the first stage, infra-red radiation is emitted and in the third stage, the characteristic yellow light emerges. This is a very common effect when gases or vapours are excited by light or other radiation.

In the case of certain solids, we may have a mixture of processes occurring. The incident light may be absorbed, resulting in the production of excited atoms, which again may return to normal in several stages. The first stage of the return may not give out radiation but may simply produce heating of the

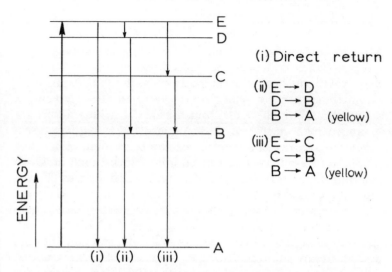

Fig. 4.4 We can represent the excited states of atoms by horizontal lines whose distance above line A, representing the normal ("ground") state, denotes the amount of energy they possess. The sodium atom can absorb ultra-violet radiation, which causes the normal atoms to change to excited ones, represented by level E. They may return to the normal state in three possible ways: E → A, E → D → B → A and E → C → B → A.

crystal. The second stage may produce light. Thus if a crystal of ruby is illuminated by blue or green light, we see a deep red fluorescence. In other cases a much more complex behaviour obtains. The atoms may return from their excited states through many stages, some of which produce heating and others light or other radiation. Many materials of this kind are used as laser crystals and will be discussed in later chapters.

The above discussion is concerned with what happens in an essentially "perfect" crystal of material. If there are structural imperfections in the crystal (e.g. due to inclusions or holes, or to the effects of strain in the material), then light may simply be scattered by them, as sunlight is scattered by dust. In this case, no changes occur in the state of excitation of the atoms in the crystal. In dealing with crystals for lasers, however, such scattering processes may nevertheless be important because they result in loss of energy from a light beam passing in one direction through the crystal.

Special effects in crystals

Most of our discussion so far has been concerned with what happens when radiation interacts with atoms—it has dealt mainly with the behaviour of the atoms as individuals. In addition to these effects, we can observe changes in the behaviour in a light beam which result from the way in which atoms are arranged in a crystal. A crystal consists of a regular three-dimensional array of atoms, which can be thought of as being made up of a pile of identical building blocks, each of which contains an identical group of atoms. In some crystals, the individual building block has the shape of a cube: this is the case for sodium chloride (common salt), copper and iron. Sometimes the building block will be rectangular, with different spacings along the three edges, as in iodine, calcium chloride and antimony sulphide. In other cases, the block may not be rectangular but have angles other than 90°, as in the case for anthracene, illustrated in Fig. 4.5. There is a whole variety of different shapes of basic block which, when repeated in all directions, represents the actual crystal.

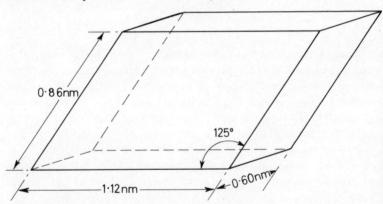

Fig. 4.5   Shape of individual cell in crystal of anthracene. (One nm (nano-metre) is a thousand-millionth of a metre.)

Let us examine what effect the crystal regularity will be expected to have on a light beam passing through the crystal. If we consider first the cubic crystal, we shall expect that whatever happens to the light, on traversing the crystal, the same effect

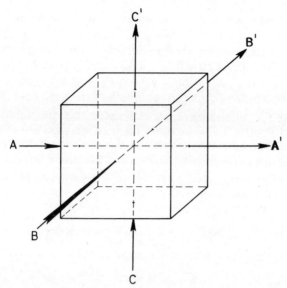

Fig. 4.6   Cubic crystals behave the same way for light travelling in the directions shown (and, indeed, for all directions).

will be observed whether the light goes along AA', BB' or CC' in Fig. 4.6. This is indeed what is found. For example the speed with which the light passes through the crystal is the same in these three directions. In fact, we find that the speed of light in cubic crystals is the same in *all* directions. In contrast, we should not expect that the crystal formed of a rectangular repeat unit would behave in the same way for all directions, and again this is what is found. The speed of light in such a crystal depends on the direction of the light beam.

Let us now recall the description we gave of a light beam in Chapter 2. This was seen as a combination of oscillating electric and magnetic fields, with the electric and magnetic oscillations perpendicular to one another. In fact, if we were able to detect the directions of the electric and magnetic fields in the light from any ordinary source, we should find that the directions of these fields varied extremely rapidly as time passed. Instead of remaining in one direction, they change in an irregular way; so that, even when looked at for a very short time, the electric and magnetic fields point in all directions around the direction of light travel. Such a light beam is termed *unpolarised*. In some circumstances, we are able to modify a light beam so that the oscillating electric field of the beam remains always in the same direction. (So does the magnetic field, which is always perpendicular to the electric field.) This may be done, for example, by reflecting the beam from a glass surface at a particular angle —the Brewster angle. Although much of the light goes into the glass, the reflected part is found to have its electric field confined to the direction shown in Fig. 4.7. Such a beam is termed *plane polarised*. Our interest in this lies in the fact that crystals may sometimes produce odd effects on beams of polarised light and that we make very good use of these effects, not only in the design of lasers but also in their application.

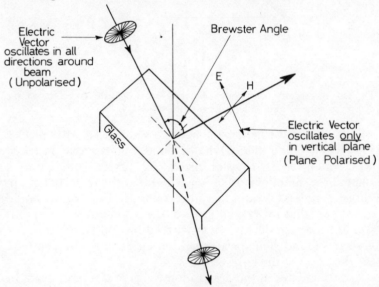

Fig. 4.7 The electric vector in the light reflected from a surface at the Brewster angle oscillates only in the direction shown.

An alternative method of producing plane polarised light is by the use of polaroid sheet—a material whose crystals allow light polarised in one direction to pass through but which absorbs light polarised in the perpendicular direction. (The effects of polarisation due to reflection can be very easily seen by looking through a piece of polaroid at the light reflected by, e.g., a polished floor, or a window. On rotating the polaroid about the viewing direction, the reflected light is seen to be alternately dimmed and passed by the polaroid. If the angle of reflection from a glass plate is right—about 52°—then the reflection can be completely stopped by the polaroid.)

If, now, we send a beam of plane polarised light through certain crystals (e.g. a quartz crystal) we find that, although the light emerging from the crystal is still plane polarised, the direction of the polarisation has been twisted from its original direction. This phenomenon—optical activity—results from the particular way in which the atoms in the quartz crystal are arranged. (In fact, we can understand how—knowing the arrangement of atoms in the crystal—optical activity must result. We may turn this argument backwards, and say that, if we observe optical activity, the atoms must be arranged in a certain way.)

This is an interesting effect but there is another, related effect which we are able to use in a very powerful way in the application of lasers. There are certain crystals which may be persuaded to produce a rotation of the direction of the electric field of a light beam if we apply a steady electric field to the crystal. Thus a crystal of potassium dihydrogen phosphate will allow a plane polarised beam of light to pass through unchanged but will cause a rotation of the plane of polarisation if a voltage is applied across the crystal. This is illustrated in Fig. 4.8. When a voltage

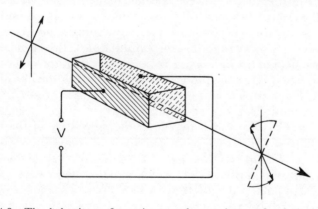

Fig. 4.8   The behaviour of certain crystals to a beam of polarised light changes when a voltage is applied across the crystal. The direction of the electric vector in the light beam is rotated from its initial direction.

is applied in this way, the crystal becomes optically active. The amount of rotation of the direction of the electric field in the light waves depends on the voltage applied. If we apply the appropriate voltage, we can arrange that the electric field of the light wave is rotated by 90°. This leads us to the interesting possibility that we may be able to control the intensity of a light beam by applying a voltage to a crystal. For suppose we place such a crystal between two polarisers which are arranged so that no light will pass. The first allows light with the electric field in, say, vertical direction to pass, while the second will let through only light whose electric field is horizontal. If, now, we apply a voltage to the crystal so that the light emerging from the crystal has its field in the horizontal direction, then while the voltage is applied to the crystal, the light beam will pass right through the system. As soon as the voltage is switched off, the light from the crystal is stopped by the second polariser. We are able to arrange voltage pulses, for application to the crystal, of very short duration and so are able to produce light flashes of very short duration. We shall see, in Chapter 11, how this effect may be applied in certain laser systems.

What happens if the voltage which we apply is not precisely the value to cause a rotation of the direction of the electric vector, so that plane polarised light emerges from the crystal? In this case, we would find (if we could devise a way of actually seeing the direction of the electric field of the transmitted wave) that the electric field of the light wave moved steadily round the viewing direction, becoming alternately stronger and weaker as time went by. If we represent the amplitude and direction of the electric field of the light wave by an arrow, then the end of the arrow would trace an ellipse, when viewed along the line of the beam (Fig. 4.9). This is termed *elliptically polarised light*. Under some conditions, it can be arranged that the ellipse becomes a circle, so that the arrow depicting the amplitude of the field maintains a constant length, but the end moves in a circle, giving us *circularly polarised light*. We must however distinguish this from unpolarised light, which we discussed earlier. In a beam of unpolarised light, the end of the arrow also moves over a circular path but it does *not* move round regularly. The end of the arrow will always be on a circle but it will dodge about from point to point in a random fashion. In circularly polarised light

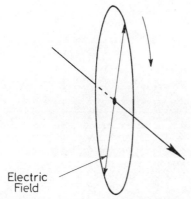

Fig. 4.9 Representation of elliptically polarised light. The end of the vector representing the electric field moves around an elliptical path.

the end of the arrow, representing the electric field of the light wave, moves smoothly and steadily around a circle—in either a clockwise or an anticlockwise direction.

Some crystals will behave in this way of their own accord, while others may be made to act on a light beam in this fashion by the application of a voltage to the crystal. We may mention in passing yet another class of materials which may be modified so that they affect a polarised light beam by the application of a magnetic field, instead of by the electric field produced by a voltage on the crystal.

In our discussion so far we have stressed that the effects on the polarisation of a light beam leading to the production of rotation of polarisation, or of elliptic polarisation, arise from the arrangement of atoms in a crystal, either in the natural state or as a result of persuasion by the application of a voltage to a crystal. In fact there are also liquids in which the latter phenomenon—modification by an applied voltage—can be obtained. In the normal way, we imagine a liquid as a collection of atoms or molecules which are not firmly located in fixed positions, as in a solid, but are free to wander around in all directions. Most liquids (although not all) have no effect on the polarisation of a light beam but there are some which, when a voltage is applied across them, do have an effect. The device shown in Fig. 4.10, termed a Kerr cell, will produce elliptically polarised light from a plane polarised beam, in much the way

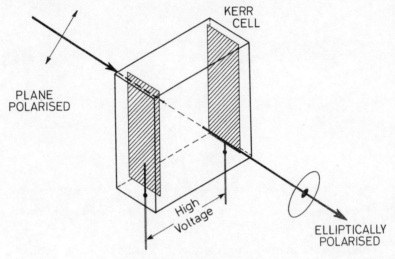

Fig. 4.10   The Kerr cell. When a voltage is applied, incident plane polarised light emerges from the cell as elliptically polarised.

that certain crystals do. With just the right voltage applied in the appropriate direction, such a cell may produce circularly polarised light, or may produce rotation in the direction of the polarisation of an incident beam.

We shall see in Chapter 11 how use is made of these effects in laser systems for the production of extremely intense light pulses—light pulses of intensities incomparably higher than have ever been produced by man, and capable of vaporising any known material.

Before concluding this chapter, we refer again to the spectrum emitted by the sun and in particular to the fact that this is found to be crossed by large numbers of very fine dark lines. If the positions of these lines are carefully measured, it is found that they correspond exactly to the positions of emission lines from a wide range of materials. Thus fine absorption lines are seen in exactly the positions of many of the lines given out by a hydrogen discharge tube. In the latter, the spectrum is seen as a set of *bright* lines against a *dark* background: in the solar spectrum, corresponding *dark* lines are seen against a *bright* background. We want to examine this phenomenon because it illustrates one of the processes which occurs when light passes through a gas. This process is of great importance for the operation and understanding of the gas laser.

The reason for the apparently strange behaviour of the sun's spectrum is easily understood if we remind ourselves of just what the sun is like. The interior of the sun is known to be extremely hot, the result of an enormous generation of energy through nuclear processes. Since the heat can most easily be lost from the surface, this part will be much cooler than the interior. It is still, however, so hot that it gives out a continuous spectrum, like that of any hot body, with a distribution of energy over different wavelengths given by a Planck curve, as discussed in Chapter 3. Now we know that on Earth, the higher we go above ground, the cooler the air becomes. Although the sun is not a solid sphere like the earth, the same applies, so that above the "surface" of the sun we expect to find cooler gas—so cool that we do not see it glowing, as we see the gas in the interior of the sun. What will we expect to happen to the light from the sun's interior as it passes through the cooler gas surrounding the central, very hot portion? Light energy of all wavelengths is present in abundance, *including* that corresponding to the amount required to raise the atoms in the cool layers to excited states. We do need to have *exactly* the right amount of energy to produce excited states of atoms in a gas in this way—too little or too much energy will not do. So some of the light from the hot region of the sun is intercepted by atoms in the cool region—but *only* at wavelengths corresponding to lines associated with atoms in that region.

At first sight, this appears a satisfactory and straightforward explanation of this effect although one further step "restores the status quo"* and may make the explanation less convincing. For the excited atoms formed may well return to their ground state and give out precisely the radiation which they absorbed. This would surely put us right back where we were? This is in fact not so because the atoms concerned have a poor memory. During the brief period in which they dither, before changing back to their normal state, they forget how they became

*Nature and Nature's laws
 Lay hid in night.
 God said "Let Newton be"
 and all was light.

It did not last.
The Devil, howling "Ho!
Let Einstein be",
Restored the status quo.

excited, which in this case was by absorbing light from the sun's interior. Now this light, which we are observing from earth (or elsewhere) travels through the cool outer gas *in one direction*. The outer gas atoms absorb some of this energy, at the precise wavelengths corresponding to the particular atom and then, on re-emission, scatter the absorbed light in all directions. Thus some of the light which was on its way to us—and which would have given us a truly continuous spectrum—is sent off in other directions and very little of it reaches us. There will therefore be dark lines in the spectrum at just those wavelengths which the atoms in the outer parts of the sun can absorb. The dark lines are known as Fraunhofer lines.

When such lines were first observed their wavelengths were carefully measured and it was found that these could generally be identified exactly with the lines emitted from many known elements, thus indicating the presence of these elements on the sun. There were however a few lines which stubbornly refused to correspond to the emission lines of any known materials. The keyword is "known". The mystery lines were assumed to belong to an undiscovered element, christened "helium". In due course, this mystery element was discovered on earth and was found to have emission lines corresponding to the unidentified Fraunhofer lines in the sun's spectrum. It may thus fairly be claimed that this element was discovered on the sun before it was found on earth.

CHAPTER FIVE

But is light really waves?

Most of the matters concerning light so far discussed in this book can be very simply accounted for in terms of the description of light as an electromagnetic wave, as described in Chapter 3. In order that we can discuss the behaviour of a laser, however, we must examine a little more closely the implication of some of the arguments used earlier, particularly in relation to the absorption and emission of light by atoms. We must also consider one or two effects which cannot readily be fitted into our picture of light as an electromagnetic wave.

Towards the end of the nineteenth century it was observed that in certain circumstances, a beam of light could cause electrons to be emitted from a metal surface: the electrons are termed photoelectrons. On our earlier description, we have no need to be surprised at this. We have been able to account for many features of the behaviour of matter by assuming that atoms can absorb energy from a light wave and become excited. In terms of our picture of an atom as a planetary system, with the nucleus at the centre and the electrons in orbits about the nucleus, we can interpret an excited atom simply as one in which the electrons have moved into a different orbit, with higher energy. Surely, then, if the light wave can give *enough* energy to the electron, it will be able to kick it right out of the atom? Fine, but it is when we measure the energy with which the photoelectrons leave the metal, and try to relate this to the intensity of the light beam, that we run into trouble. We should expect that an intense light beam would cause the photoelectrons to be emitted with more energy than would a weak beam. This does not happen: increasing the intensity of the light beam produces *more* electrons but *not* more energetic ones.

The curious feature here is that, when we look at any kind of wave motion—sound waves, seismic waves, waves on water —we always find that the amount of energy that a wave carries along is very simply related to the amplitude of the wave, being proportional to the square of the amplitude. In the case of a light wave causing photoelectrons to be emitted, it is not in the least clear why a weak beam of light produces a small number of electrons with a particular energy while a more intense beam produces more electrons *of the same energy*. However, we may well have the feeling that there is some way round this difficulty. Let us look, then, at a further feature of the photoelectric effect for which any explanation would appear to have to be very far-fetched, if couched in terms which we have been using so far.

Suppose we set up a photoelectric experiment in such a way that we can weaken the intensity of the light beam to a very low value—perhaps by putting a filter in the beam. Then, as we should expect, the weaker the beam, the smaller the number of electrons emitted each second. Imagine now that we have adjusted the light intensity so that we get one electron per second from the surface. (These will be found all to have the same energy.) Now suppose that we put in a filter which transmits only one tenth of the light falling on it. We should expect then to get one electron every ten seconds. We must, however, expect that the first electron to be emitted will come out ten seconds after we switch the light on. We expect this because the electron emitted is found to have as much energy as the light beam carries to the surface in ten seconds. In fact, we are quite likely to get an electron hopping out of the surface as soon as the light is switched on, even though the intensity is so low that it should take a long time for it to bring to the surface the amount of energy with which the electron left the surface. This worries us considerably because one of the cornerstones of modern scientific thought is that energy cannot be created—the total amount of energy (which may be in the form of mass) is always found to be constant. The balance sheet is strict—if energy appears in one place, an exactly equal amount must have disappeared from somewhere else.

The photoelectric experiments described above do in fact appear to be toppling the hallowed monument of the conservation of energy. Let us look again at the results of the weak-beam experiment and see whether our observation will in fact bear the interpretations which we have put on them. There is no problem with the electron—we can actually measure its energy. We must, however, be rather careful in what we say about the light beam. We have used the idea that light shows wave-like behaviour—and there is plenty of evidence for this. But we have *not* actually measured the amplitudes of the light beams used. We may have measured the intensity—with some kind of detector—of an intense beam and then sent the beam through a set of filters. By the time we get to the low intensities mentioned above, we find that we cannot obtain a steady reading of the intensity of the light. Thus we cannot claim that we *know* that our feeble light beam has the kind of wave property which we associate with intense beams. Given that we must of necessity modify the ideas which lead to so unequivocal a conflict with energy conservation, we do this in the simplest way possible. The fact that an electron pops out before a *continuous* wave could have brought sufficient energy means that we are wrong in assuming that the light wave *is* continuous. In fact, when we observe photoelectrons emitted by a weak beam, they do not emerge at a regular rate, but at highly variable intervals. This is almost as if the light beam consisted of a succession of particle-like entities, capable of knocking electrons out of metals.

There is one further feature to examine, namely how the above arguments apply for light of different wavelengths. (The arguments given above refer to light of a single wavelength.) Two observations are made, namely:

1 No photoemission occurs if the wavelength is too long, and
2 where photoemission occurs, the energy of the electron emitted increases as the wavelength of the illuminating beam is reduced, that is, it increases with frequency v, since v = velocity ÷ wavelength.

A study of these and many other features of the way in which light behaves leads us to the conclusion that, when light beams interact with anything so that light energy is transferred, transfer takes place only in fixed amounts and *not as a continuous stream.* The fixed amounts are referred to as light quanta, or photons, and the amount of energy in one depends on frequency, according to the relation

$$\text{Energy quantum} = \text{Planck's constant} \times \text{frequency}$$
$$E = h \times v$$

One of the reasons why we are not conscious of the quantum nature of light in everyday life is that the size of an individual light quantum is extremely small. If you stand 100 m away from a sodium street lamp the number of sodium light quanta which enter your eye every second is about three hundred thousand million. In almost every situation in which we use light sources in normal life, the number of quanta involved are enormous—we are no more conscious of the fact that light consists of a stream of quanta than we are that the tiniest particle we can see contains an enormous number of atoms.

Although the idea of light quanta having a fixed amount of energy which depends on the wavelength may appear strange at first, it becomes less so when we look back at some of the matters referred to earlier. We remarked that the wavelengths of the lines emitted by, e.g., a mercury lamp were the same for all lamps and so were clearly a characteristic of the mercury atom. We also suggested that the behaviour of atoms—either as emitters or as absorbers of light—could conveniently be discussed in terms of *excited* atoms, where the atoms have more than the normal amount of energy. Since the atom is the smallest indivisible unit of a substance (provided we do not actually break down the atom itself) and since the quantum is the smallest unit of light energy, it is not only tempting but, as it turns out, perfectly sensible to say that the excited atoms must have an excess energy of just one quantum when in the excited state.

We generally find that atoms give out lines with many different wavelengths, indicating that there must be a whole lot of different excited states. Atoms do not necessarily emit *all* their excess energy in a single quantum, in which case they would drop back to the normal, unexcited state. They may get back to normal by emitting two or more quanta. We can draw a diagram to represent this, indicating the energies of excited atoms by horizontal lines, as shown in Fig. 4.4, which represents sodium. If the sodium atom is in the level marked E, it may return directly to A, emitting ultra-violet radiation. It may come down in three stages, viz. E → D, D → B and B → A; or it may come via the route E → C, C → B, B → A. In the last two possible routes, the atom emits the familiar yellow line as it drops from level B to A. From the diagram it would appear that there are other routes—e.g., E → B, B → A or E → D, D → A. In fact we never observe radiation at a wavelength corresponding to E → B, D → A or C → A. Diagrams such as that of Fig. 4.4 are sometimes drawn with the levels displaced sideways, as in Fig. 5.1, where atoms in excited levels in any column may drop down only to levels in adjacent columns. This enables one to see at a glance, for our sodium case, that E → B, D → A and C → A will not occur.

This behaviour of excited atoms illustrates a property of light quanta which we must take note of before we endow it too specifically with the properties of a particle. This is a temptation to be resisted. Consider again the sodium atom and imagine that one such is put in the path of a beam of light (or stream of photons) with a wavelength whose energy quantum corresponds to the A → E step in Fig. 5.1. Then the sodium atom, initially

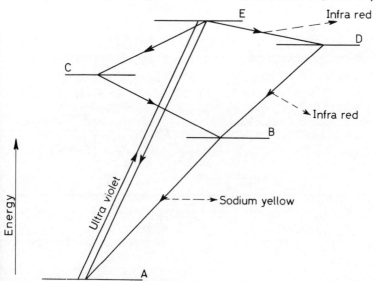

Fig. 5.1   Energy levels of the sodium atom.

with energy indicated by A, can absorb a light quantum and become excited to level E. After a very short time, the atom may decide to return to normal via the levels D and B. In so doing, it emits three light quanta, two of which have wavelengths in the infra-red and the third of which is the usual sodium yellow line. Thus we started with a single ultra-violet quantum and have ended up with three quanta, all of smaller energy. We should indeed find that the sum of the energies of the three quanta was exactly equal to that of the ultra-violet one, so that our sacred law of conservation remains inviolate. However, it is clear that the photon cannot be regarded as a particle in the sense of having a permanent identity.

In the above situation, the sodium atom *may* decide to return to normal by emitting a single ultra-violet quantum. Although the time for which the atom remains excited is very short (say a hundred millionth of a second) its memory is even shorter. By the time it changes back and lets fly its quantum, it has completely forgotten which way the incoming photon was coming. The atom may throw the photon out in any direction and the overall effect may appear as though the incoming photon had been bounced off the atom (Fig. 5.2). However, we must not

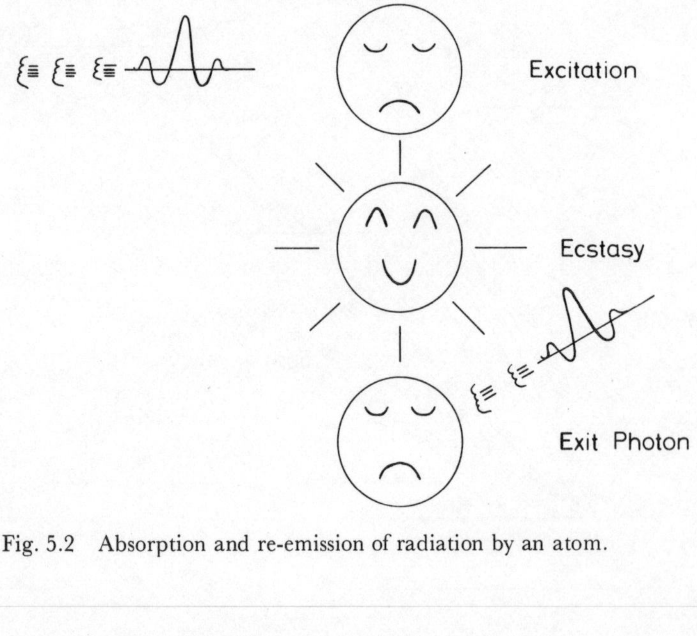

Fig. 5.2   Absorption and re-emission of radiation by an atom.

ignore the fact that, for a short period during the process, an excited atom was produced: the atom did not stay in its normal state during the bouncing operation. This is an extremely important *caveat*: if we ignore this, we exclude the possibility that someone, by acting quickly enough, may get at the atom while it is in the excited state. We shall see that the operation of a laser depends entirely on an action of this kind.

In cases where the appropriate interference with the excited atoms in a volume of gas does not occur, the light (or radiation) emitted streams in all directions. The spirit of isolationism prevails among the atoms. They become excited—e.g. by absorbing light quanta or by being struck by electrons—and each of them emits in any direction it thinks fit, regardless of what is going on around and regardless of the way in which it originally became excited. Thus the light quanta stream out in all directions and at times quite independently of one another— a process termed "spontaneous emission". In the next chapter, we shall examine another form of emission, which occurs when the excited atom is persuaded to push out its photon without our waiting for it to emit spontaneously.

The photoelectric effect is one of many which can only be sensibly described by the assumption that radiation can exchange energy only in quanta. There are many other experiments which require such a description, but which are of no concern to us in the context of a study of lasers. Suffice it to say that the notion of light quanta is now a well-established one.

Before closing this chapter, we must look at what appears as a contradiction in our description of light. It has often been said that no one could for a moment doubt the wave-like character of light on seeing interference patterns such as that of Plate 2. Such patterns can be simply and elegantly accounted for in terms of waves, which interfere so that their effects reinforce at the bright rings or fringes (Plate 2) or cancel in the regions of low intensity. This picture works so well that we must be alarmed at the prospect of replacing it with one based on the idea that light shows a particle-like behaviour. Granted that, in view of our discussion of the impermanence of quanta, we do not picture quanta as simple particles: nevertheless, it is not clear how quanta can display wave-like properties. One short answer is that *a* quantum does not exhibit wave-like properties.

It could hardly do this since it is the smallest "light-particle" that we can have. The characteristic of a wave is that it is something which varies smoothly and rhythmically, as does the height of water when waves pass over it. With the quantum, it is either there (all of it) or not. Since light beams which are intense enough to show interference effects *do* exhibit wave-like properties, we must conclude that whole collections of quanta can combine to produce a wavelike result: and that, although we cannot observe it in an individual quantum, quanta have a wave character associated with them.

We briefly mentioned the idea of *coherence* of a light wave, in the introductory chapter. On the electromagnetic description of light we know that a light wave involves an oscillating electric field. If, on sitting beside a light wave with an instrument which will measure the electric field of the wave, we found that the field oscillated perfectly regularly, as shown in the Fig. 5.3, and

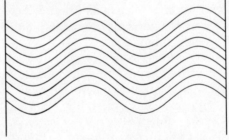

Fig. 5.3   A coherent wave. Oscillations over all parts of the wave are in step with one another.

if we moved across the light beam and still found the same regular behaviour, we should describe this as a perfectly coherent wave. We cannot do this experiment with a light wave but we can with a radio wave. For waves used for broadcasting we should find that they are coherent—that they reach their peaks and troughs at exactly regular intervals for as long as we watched. (Strictly this is true only if no programme is being broadcast.) Although we cannot view a light wave directly in this way, we have considerable evidence to show that the light from any normal source is *not* coherent. What we would expect to see, on "watching" the variations of electric field, is as if an enormous number of waves were rushing by, each lasting for only a short time, and with the peaks of the different waves arriving at completely random intervals. Fig. 5.4 gives a general idea of what would be expected. Such a wave is described as *incoherent*. For a coherent wave we know that, if the time interval between successive peaks is T, then if we get a peak at a given instant, we shall have peaks again at $T, 2T, 3T \ldots$

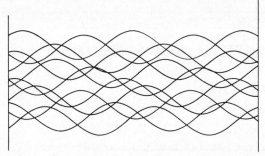

Fig. 5.4   Incoherent radiation. Although the waves in different parts have the same wavelength, they are not in step with one another. Moreover the relative phases of the waves in different parts change irregularly with time.

for as long as the wave is passing. For an incoherent wave, this will not be so. We may get a short interval with peaks arriving regularly, but after this the regularity will be interrupted.

This erratic behaviour of the light from an ordinary source does not surprise one in view of the earlier discussion on the way in which atoms emit radiation. If we generate excited atoms by passing a current through a tube of gas and if the atoms give out quanta at irregular intervals, then we should not expect perfect regularity in the pattern of light emitted. Everything fits—the whole process is an irregular one and we are not surprised. Surely, however, we have a feeling that it must be possible to organise the process? Can we not somehow persuade the atoms to emit in such a way that the resultant wave *is* coherent?

The marching army is required to break step when crossing a bridge, for fear of the destructive consequences of a perfectly regularly applied impulse to the bridge. In some ways, the achievement of co-operation between light-emitting atoms—as happens in the laser—can result in just as dramatic consequences.

CHAPTER SIX

Einstein and stimulated emission

Although the name of Einstein is associated most directly with the theory of relativity, he made significant contributions in other fields, including the photoelectric effect. In 1917, he described the way in which light (or radiation) and atoms would react on one another and provided all the fundamental information needed for the birth of the laser. In fact thirty-eight years elapsed before the first device (the maser—see Chapter 7) was constructed which made use of the principles laid down by Einstein. The laser followed some five years later.

It is interesting to speculate on the question why the realisation of the maser and laser took so long after the discovery of the underlying principles: for the direct consequence of these principles is that it is possible, if the right conditions are established, that radiation will grow in intensity as it passes through matter. There is no indication that Einstein realised that this followed from his arguments—at least nothing appears to have been written to this effect. In 1922, however, Tolman remarked that this was indeed a consequence of Einstein's theory, but gave no indication that he felt that there was anything particularly interesting about this. In 1951, Fabrikant stated quite explicitly that a population inversion should lead to wave amplification. He suggested methods of achieving a population inversion.

In the early 1950s, there appears to have been more direct interest in the possibilities of amplification which follow from the theory. There seems to be some uncertainty as to whether one can attribute specifically to an individual the precise idea which led to a working system: in times of such intensive activity this is often not possible, and the arguments which seek to establish individual credit sometimes seem petty and un-edifying. There is, however, no doubt whatever about the man —C. H. Townes—who succeeded in constructing the first device. Although differing in some features from the laser (for the device worked in a very high-frequency radio region) the maser is certainly the first device based on Einstein's predictions. (We shall discuss this device in Chapter 7.) Before we do this, let us look rather closely at the way radiation behaves.

Suppose we have an oven which has been heated to a parti-cular temperature and left long enough for the air inside to warm up to the temperature of the oven walls. Now we know how the energy of the radiation in the oven is distributed among different wavelengths. (We could find this by making a small hole in the side of the oven and by examining the radiation streaming out. If the hole were sufficiently small, it would scarcely disturb things.) The form of curve representing the radiation at different wavelengths is simply the Planck curve, already shown in Fig. 3.1.

What exactly is going on in the oven? Radiation is streaming out of the walls of the oven (and back into them again) but it may well interact with the atoms of air in the oven. The atoms may absorb radiation and become excited, as described in Chapter 4. Shortly after becoming excited they will sponta-neously emit their excess energy. There will clearly be a balance achieved between absorption and emission processes when everything has become steady.

Without knowing anything about the Planck curve, we can calculate—using what we know about the way atoms behave— the manner in which the radiation energy should vary with wavelength (or frequency). If we assume

  1 that atoms become excited by absorbing radiation,
  2 that they emit their excess energy spontaneously, and
  3 that everything has become steady,

then we are led inexorably to the curve shown in Fig. 6.1 for the energy/frequency curve. This is quite unlike the curve we obtain on measuring the radiation. It predicts, for example, that

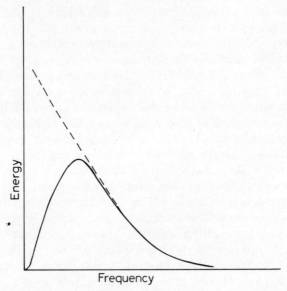

Fig. 6.1   If only spontaneous emission is taken into account, theory gives the curve marked by the dashed line. Experimentally, the full curve is obtained.

all hot bodies will emit more blue light than red. If theory and experiment disagree (provided of course there is nothing faulty about the experiment) the theory is clearly wrong. Why? The answer turns out to be very simple. We have taken account of the fact that unexcited atoms may absorb radiation and become excited. We have allowed for the fact that excited atoms change back to normal through spontaneous emission. We have *not* taken account of the fact that the excited atoms may be affected by the radiation. In spite of the fact that light-emitting atoms remain excited for only a short time, it is essential to allow for the possibility of their being acted on by the radiation present.

What does happen in this case? Does the atom absorb more energy and become even more highly excited? No—if this is assumed, then again the wrong curve is obtained. Einstein showed that the calculations agree with the radiation measurements if it is assumed that the radiation causes the excited atom to return to the normal state—or to a less highly excited state.

When the atom changes from an excited to a lower state, the

excess energy is given out as radiation. This immediately suggests the possibility of amplification, for if radiation passing through a region containing excited atoms persuades them to release their excess energy we end up with more radiation than we had at first. One important feature of the radiation given out as a result of the effect of incoming radiation on the atoms is that the direction of the induced radiation is the same as that of the incoming beam. Thus if, as in Fig. 6.2, we have a narrow beam of radiation passing into a region containing (only) excited atoms, then the beam will be amplified. The process whereby atoms may be de-excited by radiation is termed *stimulated emission*, providing two of the letters in the acronym "laser".

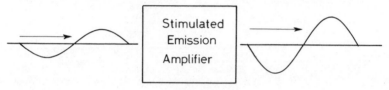

Fig. 6.2 When a beam of radiation is amplified by a stimulated emission device, it continues in the same direction.

If we can produce a box containing *only* excited atoms—that is with no lower-energy ones—then we *may* be able to extract all their excess energy into the amplified beam. Or, we may be only partially successful. The reason for this lies in the length of time for which atoms remain excited before emitting spontaneously. If this is long enough, our incoming beam of radiation may stimulate all the excited atoms to emit before they have a chance to emit spontaneously. If, on the other hand, the time in the excited state is short, many atoms may radiate spontaneously before the incoming beam can act on them. What happens depends on the frequency of the radiation concerned. If we are in the radio-frequency region the former condition applies and we can forget about spontaneous emission. The atoms remain excited long enough for them to be practically all de-excited by the effects of the normal radiation present. If, however, the radiation is around the visible region, a considerable amount of spontaneous emission occurs (Fig. 6.3.). In this case the time which the atoms spend in the excited state is

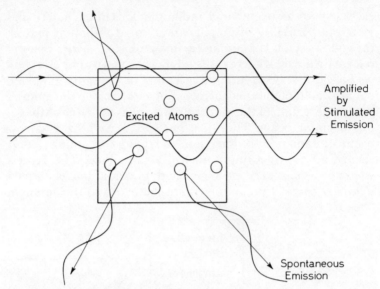

Fig. 6.3   For radiation in the visible region, some of the excited atoms in the amplifier decay by spontaneous emission.

very short. The chances of their being de-excited by radiation is very small—they almost all return to lower states through spontaneous emission.

In many situations, we are not able to produce a box containing excited atoms only. There is generally a mixture of the two, so we must consider what will happen if we send a beam of radiation through such a mixture (Fig. 6.4). Let us ask how the intensity of the beam which has passed through the mixture is affected. For the moment, ignore the effects of spontaneous emission and concentrate on the two other processes which can occur, namely absorption and stimulated emission. Each time an atom in the lower state absorbs a radiation quantum, the transmitted beam will be weakened by this amount. Each time an excited atom is stimulated to emit, the transmitted beam is strengthened—again by the energy of one quantum. What will be the overall effect? This clearly depends on whether there are more atoms present in the excited state than in the lower state. If there is an excess of lower state atoms, the transmitted beam will be weakened: if the excited atoms dominate the beam will be amplified. This seems to be a very simple condition to

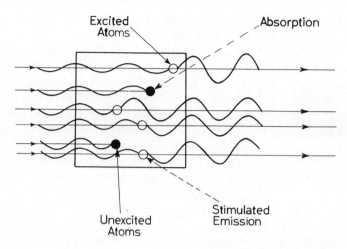

Fig. 6.4 If both excited and unexcited atoms are present, the excited ones amplify and the unexcited ones absorb radiation in the beam.

establish—more atoms in a highly excited state than in a lower one—and it is a necessary key for the release of energy in the form of a laser beam. By hindsight, we are now certain that in many of the discharges in gases which were worked on in the second and third decades of this century, such conditions must have existed. Certainly some of the results—at first sight strange ones—obtained by Ladenburg in 1932, indicate that this unusual situation must have existed in his experiments. Unusual because under very many conditions, we know that there are always *fewer* atoms in highly excited states than in lower ones.

It is just conceivable that the laser could have been discovered by sheer accident, twenty years or more before it finally appeared. With certain of the lasers now in use, all the necessary ingredients were, in fact, available thirty years ago. However, since the role of stimulated emission in causing amplification had not been realised, it was unlikely that experiments would have been made which would lead to the laser. It is, however, possible that spectroscopists of the time may have speculated on the prospects of getting very sharp spectral lines by putting a discharge *inside* the classic Fabry-Perot interferometer. There is some evidence that this was, in fact, tried, but with no result of interest. One can imagine the reaction of the experimenter if he had, by chance, got the right discharge conditions for laser action to occur. A more unexpected and dramatic result—of an enormously intense laser beam streaming out of the apparatus—could hardly be imagined. It is likely, however, in view of the state of theories at the time, that the correct explanation would have followed very quickly. It is perhaps not fruitful to pursue these idle speculations further although, in view of the very heavy expenditure on lasers by the military, it is tempting to ask whether an earlier discovery *would* have made any significant change in the course of history. The answer is almost certainly in the negative.

Let us return from this digression and recapitulate the essential features which lead to the possibility of harnessing the effect of stimulated emission for amplifying radiation. We shall then, in the next chapter, describe the first successful device—the maser—and then move on to the first working laser. The essential basic features are as follows:

1 By a variety of processes we may produce atoms with more than their normal amount of energy

2 Such atoms return to their normal state, either directly or in successive stages, emitting radiation in the process

3 The return of the atoms to states of lower energy may occur spontaneously or it may occur by radiation acting on the atom

4 When excited atoms are de-excited by a beam of radiation (which must be of just the right frequency) the excess energy from the atoms goes to increase the intensity of the beam of radiation

5 If atoms are present both in upper and lower energy states, those in the lower states absorb energy from a beam of radiation passing through the atoms whereas those in the upper state will amplify the beam

6 If there are more upper-state atoms than lower, the net result will be amplification of the beam

7 The radiation added to the stimulating beam is coherent, so that a smooth, regular wave becomes more intense and retains its smoothness and regularity

8 The radiation emitted spontaneously by atoms occurs independently of any radiation present, is incoherent and emerges in all directions.

CHAPTER SEVEN

The first device—the ammonia maser

In the discussion of the basic ideas leading to the possibilities of amplification of radiation, we have generally referred to the way in which atoms may be excited into states where they have more than the normal amount of energy. Precisely similar considerations apply to molecules, which consist of two or more atoms, joined together to form a stable group. They, too, may be excited—by the impact of electrons, by the absorption of radiation or by a variety of processes—and may give out radiation when they change to less highly excited states or to the normal state. Exactly as with single atoms they may be stimulated to emit by radiation. If we produce a collection of molecules in which particular excited states dominate over lower states, we can expect to be able to amplify radiation in the way described in the previous chapter. The first device in which such amplification was achieved employed molecules of ammonia as the active material. The ammonia maser not only signalled the first successful application of amplification by the use of stimulated emission, it provided a high quality amplifier for waves whose wavelength is about 1·2 cm. The latter was in itself a remarkable achievement and before we discuss the way in which the ammonia maser works, we shall spend a little time examining the general problems concerned with amplifying waves of this kind. We could start even a little further back with a few comments on the way in which the use of electromagnetic radiation for radio communication has evolved.

In the early days of broadcasting, the wavelengths of the radio waves used were of the order of hundreds or thousands of metres. Many present broadcasting stations still use wavelengths in this region. Their main characteristic is that they spread from a transmitting aerial in all directions. It is, in fact, almost impossible to send out a narrow beam of long wavelength radiation. To do this, one needs an aerial assembly whose size is very large compared with the wavelength being used. Thus although one *could*, say, use a parabolic "mirror", such as are used for radio-telescopes, the diameter would need to be tens or hundreds of kilometres across if a really tight beam were to be produced.

The feasibility of getting some directional characteristics for radio waves improves as the wavelength becomes shorter. For wavelengths of the order of a few metres, it is quite possible to obtain some degree of directionality, although even for these waves rather extensive installations would be required. The shorter the wavelength the smaller is the aerial assembly required to give a well-directed beam. Although for general, commercial broadcasting one needs the radio signals to spread in all directions, for communication between specific points (e.g. the relay towers used for microwave relays of telephone signals) the use of a narrow beam possesses many advantages. If the waves are travelling along a reasonably well-defined direction a much greater fraction of the power put into the transmitting aerial can be picked up at the receiver. There is thus a gain in efficiency over a long-wave system. There is another great advantage, to be discussed in Chapter 13, arising from the fact that for shorter wavelengths—i.e. higher frequencies—far more broadcast material can be carried along the wave than is the case of long wavelengths.

There have thus been two motivations for trying to use shorter wavelengths in communication—greater efficiency of point-to-point transmission systems and greater transmitting (or channel) capacity.

A considerable step forward in short-wave technology was made during the second world war. This grew up around the use of radio waves for detecting hostile aircraft or surface vessels —by radar. This entails, quite simply, the detection at the transmitter end of the minute part of the transmitted radiation which was reflected by the aircraft or vessel concerned. These systems involved sending out a series of short, intense pulses of radiation. By measuring the time between sending out a pulse and getting a return echo, the distance of the aircraft could easily be determined since radio-waves travel at the same speed as light waves, viz. 300,000 km/sec. However, it is of limited use merely to know the *distance* of an attacking vessel—the *direction* must also be known. This can be ascertained from a radio-wave system only if it is possible to send the radiation out in well defined directions. This, from the arguments set out above, implied the use of short wavelengths and to this end considerable development occurred during the second world war of systems using wavelengths of the order of a few centimetres. (10 cm and 3 cm were two widely used wavelengths for radar

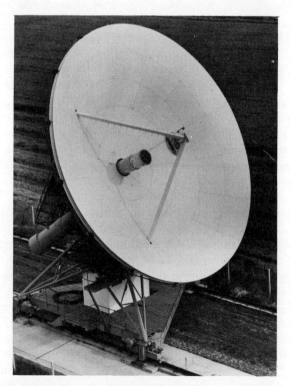

Fig. 7.1 Parabolic reflector of the type used for transmitting and receiving short-wave radio signals.

purposes.) With such a transmitter, one could fix the aerial at the focus of a large parabolic reflector (Fig. 7.1) and send out a succession of pulses while, at the same time, swinging the paraboloid around so as to "sample" whole areas of sky. Systems of this type are now commonly seen at airports or in harbours and are also carried on ships and aircraft.

When a reflected signal from a distant object—e.g. a hostile aircraft—is received, it is extremely weak and so needs to be amplified. Thus, in addition to the need for techniques for *producing* short wavelength radiation there arose the requirement that such signals could be picked up and amplified. It was in this area that there arose the subconscious yearning for something which finally took the shape of the maser. For longer wavelengths, the techniques of amplifying had used radiovalves of one sort or another. The limitation of conventional amplifiers of this type is that, in addition to performing the desired function of amplifying the waves which are fed in, they generate a whole lot of waves themselves, which become mixed up with the amplified wave itself. This effect—described as "noise"—is apparent in the ordinary radio receiver when this is tuned to a distant station and manifests itself as a rustling, hissing background like the sound of eggs frying. If the wave which is being amplified is too weak, the amplified wave is completely lost in the noise produced by the amplifier itself.

Despite enormous efforts to improve the performance of amplifiers for very short waves—those of the order of a centimetre in wavelength—the noise problem appears not to be soluble with amplifiers of the conventional, valve-based, type. It became clear that a completely new approach was required and that a system must be devised which was independent of all the conventional methods of electronics used for longer wavelengths. The maser proved to be one successful answer to this problem. In form it proved, as one might expect, to be totally different from any of the systems hitherto used for amplifying radiation

The ammonia molecule consists of four atoms, one of nitrogen and three of hydrogen, in an arrangement shown in Fig. 7.2. It possesses a vast number of possible excited states, corresponding to various complicated ways in which the atoms may vibrate around their normal positions. The details of these

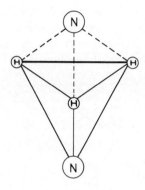

Fig. 7.2   The arrangement of atoms in the ammonia molecule. The nitrogen atom may "bounce" through the triangle of hydrogen atoms.

states need not concern us. Suffice it to say that there are two states, one of higher energy than the other and such that, when the molecule changes from the higher to the lower state, radiation of wavelength 1·2 cm is emitted. Following our earlier arguments, we see that if we can produce a larger concentration of the more energetic form of molecule than of the less energetic, we can hope to use the stimulated emission effect to amplify radiation of this wavelength.

The frequency associated with a wave of wavelength 1·2 cm is about 24,000 megacycles per second $(2·4 \times 10^{10}$ c/s). For comparison, that of the familiar sodium light is about 500 million megacycles per second $(5 \times 10^{14}$ c/s). Since the energy of a radiation quantum is equal to Planck's constant times frequency, the difference in energy for the two ammonia states is very much smaller than for the states of the sodium atom which produce the yellow sodium light. It should thus be very easy to produce excited ammonia molecules, and this is indeed so. There are even some such excited ammonia molecules in ordinary ammonia at the normal laboratory temperature. There are, however, always *more* molecules present in the lower state and the crucial problem, if we are to make an amplifier using stimulated emission, is to get rid of the lower energy molecules, so that the upper energy ones preponderate. One needs some kind of filter, which lets through only excited, and not normal molecules. This is on the face of it a difficult problem since there is really very little difference indeed between the two kinds of molecule which we wish to separate. They are the same size, so that even if we could make a mesh filter with

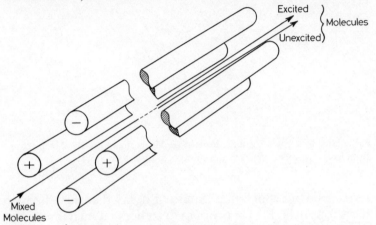

Fig. 7.3   System for focusing the ammonia molecules in the maser.

holes as small as molecules, this would not help. They behave in the same way in chemical reactions, so we cannot hope to use chemical separation. However, despite their many similarities, there is one feature in which they differ, namely in the way they behave when they are made to move through certain kinds of electric field. If we arrange four parallel rods (Fig. 7.3) and apply voltages to the rods as indicated in the diagram, then on sending a stream of mixed upper- and lower-state molecules along the centre of the system, the upper-state molecules tend to drift towards the axis whereas the lower-state molecules tend to drift in the opposite direction. If, then, we simply place a screen with a hole at the end of the system of rods, the molecules streaming through the hole will consist only of excited ones.

The excited molecules then pass into a box, or cavity, which constitutes the amplifier. A feeble signal wave is fed into one end of the cavity and an amplified wave, the result of amplification by stimulated emission from the ammonia molecules, emerges at the other end. Since waves of this wavelength (1·2 cm) fall in the microwave region of the electromagnetic spectrum, the process is described as *microwave amplification* by the *stimulated emission* of *radiation*. The initial letters of the keywords in this phrase provides the acronym "maser" used to describe the system.

In fact, the amount of amplification achieved by a wave which simply makes one passage through the box is very small. Many of the excited molecules present would not be de-excited in a single transit of the wave. The cavity is therefore made with highly reflecting walls so that radiation fed into it can make many to-and-fro reflections inside the cavity. Each time the wave passes through the cavity some emission from the excited molecules is stimulated and the wave grows in intensity.

Why is an amplifier of this type so much better than the traditional valve variety? In contrast to ordinary amplifiers, the maser generates only a minute amount of noise. For this reason, the arrival of the maser was a highly significant development in the evolution of electronic amplifiers. As mentioned above, the problem of noise in ordinary amplifiers had not been solved for existing systems and, moreover, showed no signs of being solved. An enormous amount of effort on this problem over many years had resulted in only rather small improvements. The trouble arises from a number of causes, but one recurring one in all ordinary systems is that somewhere or other a beam of electrons is used, in a valve or tube. The beam is produced by heating a wire or cathode to a high temperature, when electrons are freely given out. Although it is fairly easy to marshall the emitted electrons into a suitable order, the basic problem is that they do not all leave the cathode with the same speed. Thus instead of parading through the system like a well-drilled army, they tend to rush through rather like a rioting crowd on the move. This irregularity in their motion gives rise to the noise which causes trouble when we try to amplify very weak signals.

It will be seen from Fig. 7.4 and from the description of the maser that there is no electron beam involved, so that this source of noise is absent. Does this mean that the maser amplifier gives no noise whatever? Not quite, although the amount of noise which it does give is so small that it is extremely difficult to measure. The noise arises from an effect which we discussed in

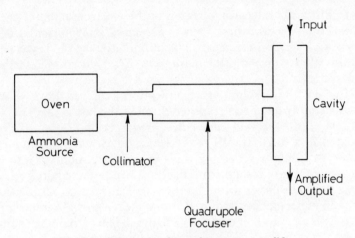

Fig. 7.4   Schematic of complete maser amplifier.

Chapter 5 but which we have not so far mentioned in our account of the ammonia maser. We know that the amplification of the maser arises from the stimulated emission of the excited molecules. We know, also, however, that excited molecules will emit spontanously if left to themselves. Moreover such spontaneous emission is independent of the presence of any waves. Any waves produced by spontaneously emitting molecules will not, except in the event of an unlikely chance, be in step with the waves which we are trying to amplify. Some of the spontaneously emitted waves will emerge from the amplifier, mixed up with the wave which we are trying to amplify but, since the unwanted waves do not combine smoothly—i.e. are not coherent—with the amplified wave, they will cause random variations in the output. These variations are nothing whatever to do with the wave which we sent into the amplifier and they constitute noise.

This effect is extremely small in the ammonia maser for a very simple reason. As seen from Fig. 7.4, the ammonia molecules are fired through the collimator, separating rods, diaphragm and cavity, finally streaming out of the cavity itself, after which they are condensed on to a cool surface. On the average, for a typical maser, the time taken by the molecules to get through the system is about 10^{-4} seconds. Now if we calculate the interval between the excitation of an ammonia molecule to the state of interest and the spontaneous emission of its excess energy, we find this to be about 10^7 seconds. (This does not mean that all molecules stay excited for this time—the times for individual molecules vary in the way shown in Fig. 7.5. It does, however, mean that the number of ammonia molecules which emit spontaneously as they go through the maser system is extremely small.)

In some respects, the ammonia maser is an almost ideal system in the sense that (1) it proves possible to arrange that only excited atoms pass into the amplifying region and (2) the effects of spontaneous emission are almost negligible. These conditions never obtain in the region of lightwaves, so that the laser is far less useful as an amplifier than the maser. We shall see, however, in the next chapter that the laser has other features of interest and importance.

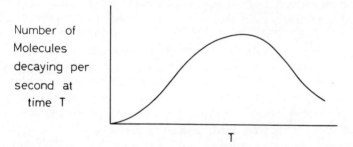

Fig. 7.5 Distribution of times for which ammonia molecules are in the excited state used in the maser.

CHAPTER EIGHT

The first laser—and its successors

Some time before attempts were made to make a working laser, Schawlow and Townes published a paper which spelled out the problems likely to be met in any maser which was to work with visible light. They also gave a possible design of a laser system and suggested materials which might be used.

This paper became a classic in a remarkably short time. Although the rapid developments which followed meant that much of the detail of the Schawlow-Townes paper was superseded and elaborated, most of the essential, core ideas were set out in this definitive contribution to the field.

Before we discuss the first successful laser, let us look at one or two of the differences between masers and lasers, in order to see where difficulties lie. In our discussion of the ammonia maser in the previous chapter we noted that the effects of spontaneous emission on the working of the maser were almost negligible. Practically all the ammonia molecules return to their lower state by stimulated emission. Since we have arranged that there is an excess of upper-state molecules, we can amplify an incoming wave and so produce a more intense beam *with very little noise* from spontaneous emission. As mentioned in the discussion in Chapter 6, for atoms or molecules which give out light, or near-visible radiation, the time spent in the excited state is extremely short—of the order a hundred-millionth of a second. Such atoms tend to return to the lower state by spontaneous emission. In fact, far from our being able to ignore spontaneous emission, we find that this is the dominant process. Certainly if we simply produce a flask of excited atoms (for example as we have in a mercury or sodium street lamp) we should find that the effects of *stimulated* emission were negligible. The atoms decay by spontaneous emission so quickly that there is hardly any time for the radiation present to get at them while they are excited, in order to produce stimulated emission. This, then, is one severe problem in moving from the radio wavelength region to the region of visible light.

A second problem concerns the ease with which we can produce excited atoms. This again depends on the wavelength involved in the emitted radiation. We noted, when discussing ammonia, that even at room temperature, there were many excited molecules present. This is because the extra energy involved is very small. In the course of colliding with one another, as the molecules bounce around in space, they can easily exchange some of their energy of motion and so produce excited atoms. When we consider atoms or molecules in excited states which have enough energy to give out visible light, the situation is very different. The energy needed to excite to these relatively high energy levels is very large compared with that available from their energy of motion. By chance, the odd atom may, through a lucky sequence of collisions, get up enough speed to be able to produce a sufficiently highly excited atom, but this occurs only very rarely. Thus in all the air lying vertically above a 100 km square on the earth's surface, we should expect to find only about a thousand such atoms—out of the 10^{41} or so atoms present. Clearly then in this case we must work fairly hard to produce enough excited atoms to be able to make stimulated emission devices work. We can do this by passing an electric current through the gas or by exposing it to a very intense source of light. In the first case, the electrons constituting the electric current have enough energy to produce excited atoms by collisions. In the second, the atoms can absorb energy from the light or other radiation and so be excited into upper states.

We still have the problem of getting an *excess* of atoms in highly excited states over those in lower energy states. This is achieved in a number of ways, which will be discussed when we come to examine in detail how typical systems work.

The first successful laser used a crystal of ruby, artificially grown. Ruby consists of a crystal of aluminium oxide in which a few of the aluminium atoms have been replaced by atoms of chromium. The normal aluminium oxide crystal—in a form known as sapphire—is a colourless material. The substitution of chromium gives the crystal the characteristic red colour of the gem stone. This colour arises from the fact that the chromium atoms in the lattice are able to absorb blue and green light, but not red, so that if we pass white light into the crystal, only the red light comes through. Thus the mere action of sending white light into the crystal produces some excited atoms. In fact, the chromium atoms sit in the ruby crystal in some of the places normally occupied by aluminium atoms and in such a way that three of their outer electrons are effectively given up to other atoms in the crystal, so we are concerned with chromium ions, rather than with ordinary (neutral) atoms.

What happens to the excited ions of chromium produced in this way? Since the excited atom or ion is an unnatural state, the atoms decay and give out their excess energy. In gases, this usually results in the re-emission of light—or of radiation of other wavelengths, in the manner described in Chapter 3. The situation in ruby is a little more involved than this. Since the chromium ions are closely surrounded by other atoms in the crystal, it is possible for some of the excess energy of the ions to be handed on to the surrounding atoms. This makes the atoms vibrate a little faster than normal—another way of saying that the crystal heats up. In ruby, only a part of the energy of the excited chromium ions is given up in this way. The result is that, after this process, the chromium ions are still excited, although with rather less energy than hitherto. At this point the chromium ions find it easier to get rid of their remaining surplus energy by giving out light—in this case in the form of a deep red emission. This process, already referred to at the end of Chapter 4, and known as fluorescence, plays a vital role in the operation of the ruby laser. The effect may be easily demonstrated by exposing a crystal to the radiation from an ultraviolet lamp. The ruby crystals glow with a rather beautiful, rich red light.

The steps involved in the fluorescent process are shown on the energy diagram in Fig. 8.1. Only the most important steps

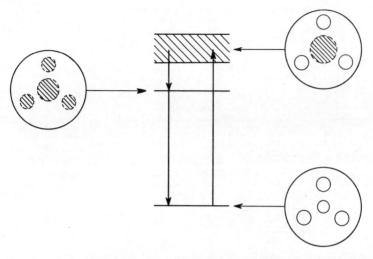

Fig. 8.1   Stages in the production of fluorescence in ruby. The centre circle represents a chromium ion. Shading indicates excitation.

are shown. Thus although some of the excited ions can drop back to the normal state by giving out all their excess energy in one go, this happens only rather rarely. Most of them return by the route shown in the figure.

If we use only a rather feeble source of light to illuminate the crystal, then at any given time we shall have only a few of the chromium ions in excited states. Most of them will be in the normal state, with only a very small fraction in the level from which red fluorescence occurs. In the hydrostatic analogy shown in Fig. 8.2(a), the "fluorescent" tank T will, for only a slow rate of pumping, contain very little water. If, however, we pump really hard, we are able to get more water into T than is left in the bottom tank (Fig. 8.2(b)). Notice that in either case, there is very little water in the top tank—the rate of flow through the large pipe into T means that the water drains into T almost as quickly as it is pumped in. The possible flow rate from T back to the bottom tank is much more restricted, so that a large volume may be pumped into T. In the ruby crystal, the chromium ions spend only a very short time in the uppermost levels, dropping immediately to the fluorescent level. From here, however, they take much longer to leak back to the normal state.

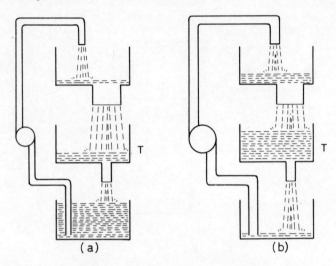

Fig. 8.2(a)   Hydrostatic analogy for feeble illumination of ruby crystal.
Fig. 8.2(b)   The situation for very intense illumination. A "population inversion" occurs between tank T and the bottom tank.

We thus have a possible way of producing an inversion of population—of getting more atoms into the excited state than in the lower state and so of fulfilling one of the conditions for amplification. However, we still have the problem that practically all of the radiation given out in the fluorescent process will be by spontaneous emission, since this is the predominant mechanism by which the ions rid themselves of their excess energy.

Imagine now that the ruby crystal, with its excited ions produced by exposing it to a brilliant light, is placed between a pair of parallel mirrors (Fig. 8.3). Many of the excited chromium atoms will give out their excess energy by spontaneous emission, in all directions and the light emitted will stream off never to return. A few of the atoms, however, will give out light in the direction of the mirrors. If the light falls squarely on the mirror, it will return through the crystal and be reflected by the mirror at the opposite end. This process will go on and on. When this radiation interacts with an unexcited chromium ion, some energy will be absorbed. If it strikes an excited ion, the radiation will be amplified. If, then, we have a population inversion,

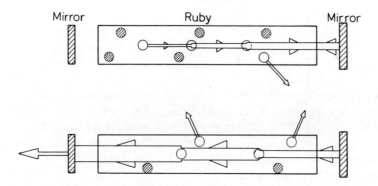

Fig. 8.3 Excited ruby in a resonator made of two parallel mirrors. As the wave passes through the ruby, it is amplified. Some of the radiation passes out through the partially transparent mirror at the left hand end.

the back-and-forth wave will on balance be amplified and will simply go on getting more and more intense.

What about the difficulty that the atoms emit spontaneously so readily, before we have a chance to produce stimulated emissions? The key here is that, if we have *enough* radiation present, we *shall* be able to de-excite the atom by the radiation, even before it decides to emit spontaneously. The chances of spontaneous emission occurring are fixed—they do not depend on how much radiation is present. The chances of producing stimulated emission increase as the intensity of radiation increases. The more radiation quanta present, the more chance there is that one of them will collide with an excited ion before spontaneous decay occurs. Since the mirror system of Fig. 8.3 leads to a continuous build-up of intensity, we are bound, sooner or later, to reach the stage where very large numbers of excited ions are contributing their excess energy to the beam.

This argument clearly applies *only* to the radiation travelling at right angles to the mirrors. For other directions, either the radiation misses the mirrors altogether or (if the initial beam strikes the mirror in a skew direction) streams out of the ruby after a few reflections. We thus have the possibility of building up an extremely intense beam of light in the direction of the axis only, and not in other directions.

If all the light falling on the mirrors is returned through the crystal, we should never know whether these things were happening unless we sat inside the crystal (although by so doing, we should get in the way, and stop the system working). We do not, however, require that the mirrors reflect *all* the light falling on them. They must reflect enough to ensure that the radiation inside the system goes on building up. Thus suppose one of the mirrors reflected only 80% of the light falling on it, but that on a round trip through the crystal the amplification of the wave amounted to 30%. There would still be a net gain, since only 20% is "lost" at the mirror, whereas 30% is gained from stimulated emission. In Chapter 4 we mentioned the use of the "one way" mirror, which reflected only part of the light falling on it, but at the same time transmitted some. Such a mirror at the end of the ruby would mean that, each time the beam inside the system struck the mirror, some of the light emerged. Since the beam inside goes on being reflected for as long as the system is working, so a continuous stream of light emerges through the mirror.

This was the basis of the first successful laser, operated by Maiman in 1960. The system was even simpler than that shown in Fig. 8.3 since the ends of the ruby rod were polished flat and parallel and were coated with a reflecting material. At one end, the coating was thin enough to permit the beam to emerge. The ruby was placed inside a helical flash-tube (Fig. 1.1) through which a large, brief pulse of current was passed. The intensity required to produce sufficient excited ions in the ruby was so high that it could not be sustained. Moreover, as noted above, some of the energy given out by the chromium ions appears as heat in the crystal. For this reason prolonged operation was not possible and the duration of the illuminating flash was restricted to about a thousandth of a second.

The result was dramatic. A brief flash of red light emerged from the end of the ruby, in the form of a pencil-like beam with a very small angular spread. This was in fact the very first time that a light source had been made with this property. Since all normal sources emit almost entirely by spontaneous decay, these sources give out light in all directions. Pencil-like beams may be produced only by auxiliary lenses, mirrors and diaphragms, and in these systems much of the light initially given out is lost. In the laser, a very large part of the light emitted comes out along the narrow beam.

The intensity of the beam emitted by Maiman's ruby was enormous. During the brief flash—lasting a few ten-thousandths of a second, the power was about 10,000 watts. Let us compare this with what happens with an ordinary light source, taking into account that an ordinary source gives out light in all directions. Maiman's ruby produced a flash of 10,000 watts and, because of the narrowness of the beam, delivered this into a spot a few millimetres in diameter at a distance of about a metre from the ruby. Compare this with, say, the power which would go through a similar area from an ordinary source emitting 10,000 watts of light. (This is in fact an enormous power for a conventional source.) Since, as seen in Fig. 8.4, the ordinary source sends its light in all directions, less than one thousandth of the light would in this case be received over the area in question. Or let us compare the familiar 100 watt lamp. Although such a lamp consumes 100 watts of electrical power, only about 10 watts of this emerges as visible light. The remainder appears partly as radiation which is outside the range of sensitivity of the human eye and partly as heat. Taking this into account, we find that the intensity of the light from Maiman's laser was more than a million times that received from the 100 watt bulb.

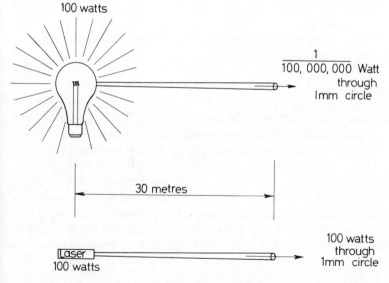

Fig. 8.4 Laser and conventional sources compared.

Thus in respect of power and directionality, even the first operating laser proved to be a remarkable source. In the subsequent development of the ruby laser, further strides in technology have led to massive further developments. The power attainable from the present (1970) generation of ruby lasers is about ten thousand *million* watts, in contrast to the ten thousand watts of the first device. It is unlikely that the output power directly from a ruby laser will go significantly higher than this for the simple reason that at such high powers, the forces acting on the atoms in the ruby crystal are approaching those at which the crystal would be torn apart. It is in fact possible to operate ruby lasers now under conditions where they damage themselves during the operation. There are, however, rather subtle techniques whereby, in spite of this limitation, even higher powers can be produced. These are referred to in Chapter 11.

The ruby laser possesses another remarkable property, distinguishing it from the normal light source. The normal fluorescent emission from a ruby crystal (not in a laser form) is in the red part of the spectrum and covers a small range of wavelength. This is rather narrower than is generally found in the fluorescence from crystals, but not as narrow as the lines emitted by an ordinary discharge in a gas. The light emitted by a ruby *laser* however is significantly sharper in wavelength than that of the ordinary material. This arises because of the way in which the light waves which are reflected back and forth in the cavity build up to form an intense pattern. We know that if we set up waves in a rope, by waggling the end, there are only certain definite wavelengths which will form a steady pattern. Similarly the organ pipe emits a sound wave of particular pitch because resonance occurs only for certain definite wavelengths. These depend on the length of the rope, pipe or other resonator. In the case of light waves between two mirrors, we can build up an intense pattern only if an exact number of waves will fit between the mirrors, as in Fig. 8.5. This means that, although the chromium ions in ruby can give out light over the band of wavelengths shown in Fig. 8.6, only certain wavelengths can be generated by the laser. The possible wavelengths depend on the distance between the mirrors (or on the length of the ruby, if the mirror coatings are put on the end-faces). If there is only one possible wavelength

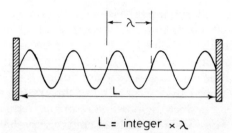

$$L = \text{integer} \times \lambda$$

Fig. 8.5 High intensity occurs only if an exact number of waves fit into the distance between the mirrors. (For light waves, there are about twenty-thousand waves to one centimetre.)

which will resonate, the laser gives out a single sharp line. If two or more wavelengths can resonate, the laser may emit two or three lines simultaneously.

The lines emitted by the laser are thus much sharper than the line which would be given by the non-lasing crystal. An important feature of the laser is that, in principle, the lines become sharper the higher the power of the output. This is in direct contrast to the way in which any ordinary source behaves. Thus if we look at the spectrum (Plate 3) of a sodium lamp of moderate power, we see sharp lines. The spectrum from a high-power lamp exhibits broader, more diffuse lines. The laser is

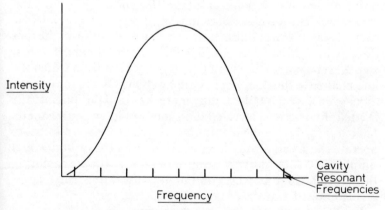

Fig. 8.6 The chromium ions in ruby give out light over the band of frequencies shown. For mirrors at the end of a ten centimetre crystal, only the frequencies indicated ("cavity resonant frequencies") will fit in between the mirrors, as in Fig. 8.5.

the only source of light or near-visible radiation which behaves in this way, giving *sharper* lines for higher power. The behaviour of ruby is a bit more involved in this respect because in order to make the ruby laser work at all, very intense illumination is necessary and the crystal gets very hot during the illuminating flash. The heating causes expansion of the crystal, so that the length changes, as does the possible resonant frequency. Thus although at a given instant, the laser emits a very sharp line, the wavelength of the line drifts about during the laser operation. We shall see that this effect is not present in the usual gas laser (Chapter 9).

Ruby seems to be an extremely good material for a laser. In addition to being able to absorb light for excitation of its chromium ions and of emitting fluorescence, it is an extremely hard, robust material, capable of withstanding rough handling, and is also chemically inert. It is only with great difficulty, how-ever, that a ruby laser can be persuaded to operate con-tinuously, instead of in brief flashes. The power at which the ruby laser works continuously is very much lower than under pulsed conditions, although still giving an intensity enormous compared with a conventional source. The basic problem with the ruby is that the atoms which produce the laser emission do so by changing from an excited state to the *normal* state. So, in order to get the inversion necessary for the laser to operate, more than half the chromium ions must be pushed up into the excited state. Now, as discussed above, we do not push the ions directly into the state from which fluorescence occurs. The first step is excitation to much more energetic states from which the ions change to the fluorescing state by giving heat to the crystal. Thus even if we put only slightly more than half the ions into the excited (fluorescent) level, all those ions would, in getting there, have dumped some heat into the crystal. If we were to try to operate the normal ruby laser continuously, the crystal would simply melt. Alternatively we must provide adequate cooling of the crystal. In this way continuously-operating ruby lasers giving about 1 watt have been constructed.

Oddly enough, the way in which ruby crystals fluoresce is somewhat unusual. It is far more common for the ions in crystals to give out fluorescence but to end up still in an excited state, after giving out their radiation. Thus in contrast

to the energy diagram of Fig. 8.1, that shown in Fig. 8.7 tends to
be more common. Now from the point of view of making a laser,
the latter type of diagram appears more attractive. Provided the
ions in the level B can get back to the normal state easily, we are
relieved of the problem of having to excite more than half the
ions in the normal state. In fact if, as generally happens (sometimes by cooling the crystal), level B stays fairly empty—which
it will do if ions drop back to the normal state very quickly—
then any ions pushed into level A will create an inversion between A and B. This has provided the mechanism of operation
of a whole range of lasers, in which small numbers of particular
atoms are put into suitable crystals as hosts.

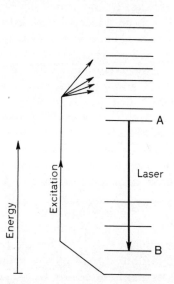

Fig. 8.7   Type of energy level distribution often found in fluorescing crystals.

One of the earliest lasers of this type involved the use of
calcium fluoride, into which small amounts of uranium were
included. The uranium atom sat in place of some of the normal
calcium atoms. This laser produced radiation in the infra-red
region of the spectrum, with a wavelength of 2·5 micrometres
(0·00025 cm). Since that time, many such systems have been
made, generally with atoms of the rare earth series as the active
material. The rare earth atoms are shown in Table 8.1. The

ones which have been successfully used in lasers are shown with an asterisk.

Table 8.1
The Rare Earth Elements

Lanthanum	Gadolinium
Cerium	Terbium
*Praseodymium	*Dysprosium
*Neodymium	*Holmium
Promethium	*Erbium
*Samarium	*Thulium
Europium	*Ytterbium

Of particular interest in the above list of elements is neodymium. This has been incorporated into many different crystals to yield lasers which give out near infra-red radiation at a wavelength of 1·06 micrometres (0·000106 cm). Two such host materials are of special interest. Yttrium aluminium garnet provides comfortable hospitality for the neodymium ion and leads to a laser which will give high power pulses (about 10^6 watts) or will work well continuously, providing an infra-red beam of about 1000 watts. The other host material is glass. It is unusual for glass to serve as a laser host, for a variety of subtle reasons, although there are many points in favour of using glass where possible. One advantage is that it is infinitely easier to make than the usual crystal materials employed. This seems to be only partly due to the fact that man has been making glass since the time of the ancient Egyptians. The growing of crystal materials is intrinsically more difficult. Extremely careful control of the conditions attending the growth of most laser crystal materials is paramount. In fact, even with the best control attainable, results cannot always be guaranteed. The possession of the necessary green fingers is at least as essential as that of sophisticated experimental equipment.

Switching from a gardening metaphor to a culinary one, we may suspect some of the developments in laser materials to have originated under a chef rather than a materials scientist. Thus the incorporation of a mixture of thulium, erbium, ytterbium and holmium in yttrium aluminium garnet leads to a very efficient laser material. The material is, appropriately enough, known as "alphabet soup". Neither vinegar nor garlic is

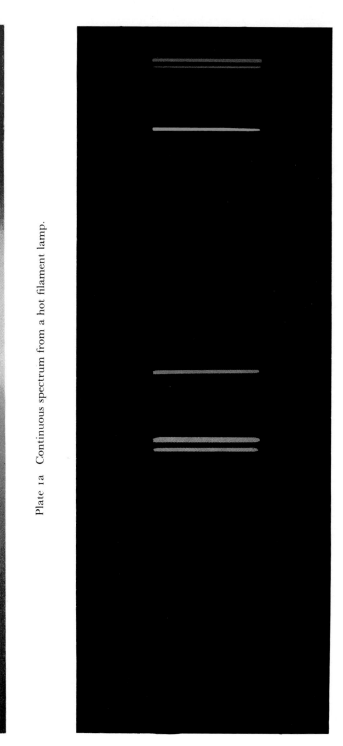

Plate 1a   Continuous spectrum from a hot filament lamp.

Plate 1b   Line spectrum from a mercury discharge lamp.

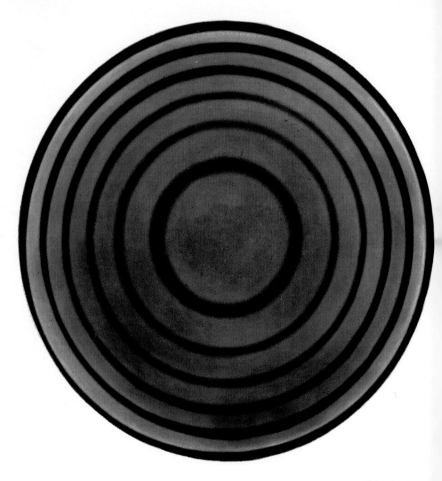

Plate 2   Newton's Rings, formed by interference of mercury green light in the space between a flat plate and a lens.

added during the preparation. The choice of materials is in fact less arbitrary than might appear at first sight. Although holmium possesses energy levels which give rise to an efficient laser line, it does not possess suitable absorption properties, so that it is difficult to obtain adequate excitation of the holmium ions. The other rare earth ions not only give the crystal suitable absorbing properties, so that excitation through illumination (with a tungsten lamp) is possible; they also are able to hand on much of their energy of excitation to the holmium ions.

Our understanding of the detailed processes going on in complex crystals of the type mentioned above is still rather limited, although it is steadily increasing. Alphabet soup illustrates a way in which considerable subtlety can be brought to bear in the design of laser materials and it is likely that new generations of laser materials will emerge from such studies.

It is interesting perhaps to reflect on the atmosphere of excitement which prevailed at the time when Maiman's work on the ruby laser was in progress. Work on lasers was almost exclusively confined to the U.S.A. and the U.S.S.R., in the former of which several groups were devoting enormous efforts towards the laser goal. Representatives of the technical press besieged the various laboratories, seeking information on progress and estimated dates at which success was to be expected. Tongue-in-cheek comments were fatal—statements such as "plans were in hand and the first laser is scheduled to work at 3.45 p.m. on a date six weeks hence" were solemnly reported and a spirit of elated competition prevailed. A flood of notes and papers explaining how a laser could be built (by someone else) poured into the editors of scientific journals, with the result that the editor of one such journal issued an edict that no further papers of this kind would be accepted. Results, not predictions, would be needed. It is therefore singularly unfortunate that, when Maiman's first report of a successful laser was submitted to the said journal, it was rejected. The editors had presumably become so accustomed to "non-result" papers that this one was swept out with the rest. There was no difficulty in finding an alternative publisher and Maiman's paper took its rightful place in a formidable and ever-increasing list, now running into many thousands of papers on this subject.

CHAPTER NINE

The gas laser

Shortly after the arrival of the ruby laser came the first laser to work with a gas as the amplifying medium. This laser involved the use of a mixture of helium and neon and provided, as did the ruby laser, a new source with remarkable properties. The mode of excitation of the gas laser was quite different from that of the ruby device, for the reasons which we now discuss.

In both gas and solid laser systems we have the common problem of producing large numbers of excited atoms or ions, together with the problem of achieving an excess population of atoms in a higher energy state than exists in a lower one. In the case of the solid state lasers described in the last chapter, we are able to obtain this excitation by exposing the crystal to a very brilliant flash of light. The light given out by the very powerful flash tubes used (or the tungsten filament lamps used for the more recent solid lasers) consists of radiation with its energy spread over many wavelengths. Thus the tungsten lamp gives out radiation roughly corresponding to the Planck curve shown in Fig. 3.1. If we pass such radiation through a low pressure gas, we find that almost all the radiation goes straight through, except for a number of very small slices, as shown in Fig. 9.1. We can see why this must be from a study of the possible energy levels for atoms in a gas. Atoms in the normal state *can* be excited to higher levels by absorbing radiation from a beam, but only if the frequency of the radiation is just right. The energy $h\upsilon$ associated with the radiation must match closely the energy

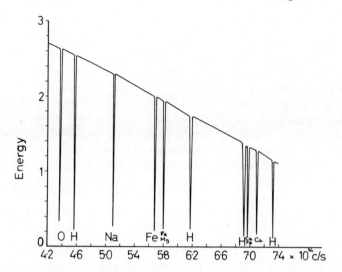

Fig. 9.1 Absorption lines occur in the light from a continuous source if the light is passed through a cool gas. The elements causing the absorption lines are shown.

required to excite the atom. Since only a small number of specific frequencies will do this, most of the radiation of the Planck type goes straight through the gas, without being absorbed and so producing excited atoms. Why is it that we can use this method for crystal lasers? The reason can be seen from Figs. 8.1 and 8.7, which show the energy levels for typical crystal materials. For some energies there are almost continuous regions of wavelength which can be absorbed by the crystal. In this case, then, a lot of energy can be absorbed from continuous sources and so large concentrations of excited atoms can be produced.

This type of excitation is for the most part not possible with gases. There is just one situation where it is—namely when there exists a gas which, when operated in a discharge tube, gives intense emission lines at exactly the right wavelength for exciting some other gas. This is the rarest of coincidences although there is one laser which has been made to operate in this way. When an intense discharge is run in helium, a very intense line is given out at a wavelength of 388·8 nm (in the near ultraviolet region). It so happens that the energy of a quantum for this radiation matches almost exactly that required to produce excited atoms of caesium. Thus if caesium vapour (obtained by heating the metal in a vacuum system) is exposed to the radiation from a helium lamp, excited atoms are produced just in the one level, corresponding to the energy of the helium quantum. The caesium atoms then return to their normal state through several intermediate transitions (Fig. 9.2). Because of the properties of excited caesium atoms, inversions of population occur in the two pairs of levels shown and laser action has been obtained at the two infra-red lines involved.

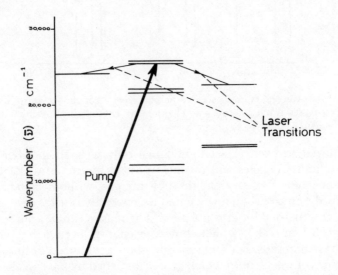

Fig. 9.2　Energy levels for caesium vapour.

It is interesting to note that, in the first paper (of Schawlow and Townes), a similar proposal was made for a system employing a mercury lamp and potassium vapour. This system has never been made to work, for reasons which are still not clear.

Thus we are for the most part denied the method of producing excited atoms of gases by absorption of light. There is, however, a simple and powerful method of exciting gas atoms to which we have often referred, namely by the passage of an electric current through the gas. The familiar neon sign and street sodium lamp are two everyday examples of this. By passing a large enough electric current through a gas, very high intensities of light can be produced. In fact this is precisely how we obtain the very high intensity flash of light required to operate the ruby laser. There are, however, advantages and disadvantages in the use of a discharge for producing excited atoms. On the one hand, very high concentrations of excited atoms can be produced in this way. On the other, the excitation is much less specific. It is not possible to arrange for any particular distribution of excited atoms, in order to obtain the inversion needed for laser action.

During 1959, Javan, working at Bell Telephone Laboratories, U.S.A., began to study the factors which govern the concentrations of atoms in different energy states where excitation is produced by collisions with electrons, as in a discharge tube. There are very many such factors, but the two important ones are

1 the rate at which electrons collide with the atoms (excited and normal), and

2 the changes of energy of the excited atoms through spontaneous emission.

The second factor depends simply on the characteristics of the atom, and so is outside the experimenter's control. The first factor depends on the number of electrons present—that is on the current flowing through the tube—and is capable of being controlled. Javan showed, in a theoretical analysis, that conditions should be attainable in which inversions of population could occur. A further development towards the evolution of a gas laser came with the realisation that the populations of some excited levels could be strongly influenced by the presence of gases which possess metastable levels. In our earlier discussions, we have described how excited atoms tend to return to their normal state by giving out their excess energy as radiation. Although this occurs very widely there are certain cases in which excited atoms cannot do this. Something in their make-up prevents them from sending out radiation and they prefer to give up their excess energy in other ways. Such atoms are termed metastable and they have the characteristic that they remain excited much longer than do atoms which can shake off their excess energy as radiation. Generally such metastable atoms will bounce around—still in their excited state—until an especially favourable opportunity arises for dumping their excess energy. One such opportunity comes when they collide with the wall of the containing vessel. Another—and this is the one of vital importance for certain lasers—is when they collide with another atom which requires practically the same amount of energy for it to become excited. If this happens, the metastable atom will drop back to its normal state and the second atom will become excited.

Helium is one of the gases which possess metastable states. Neon happens to possess excited states with energies very nearly equal to those of the helium metastables. The energy levels for these two gases are shown in Fig. 9.3. If a discharge is run in such a mixture, excited atoms (of both gases) will be produced —many of them of much higher energy than those shown in the diagram. Many of the excited helium atoms will cascade down from their high-energy states and end up on the two metastable levels shown. Since they cannot make the last step down by the easy step of giving out radiation, they wander around, somewhat frustrated, until they hit either the wall or a neon atom in its normal state. Under the conditions of interest, the helium metastables make many collisions with neon atoms in the distance travelled from the middle of a typical discharge tube to its

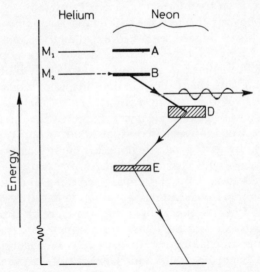

Fig. 9.3   Energy levels for helium and neon. M_1 and M_2 are metastable.

wall, so that the chance of producing excited neon atoms, in levels A or B (Fig. 9.3), is very high.

When the neon atoms in level B lose some of their energy and move to state D, they emit infra-red radiation of wavelength 1·15 micrometres (0·000115 cm). The characteristics of the neon atom are such as to make level D a slightly uncomfortable level, so they do not stay long but very quickly give out more radiation and thus end up in level E. In this circumstance, with a rapid flow of atoms into state B (from collisions of normal neon atoms with metastable helium) and a rapid flow of atoms out of state D, the conditions are right for an inversion of population between levels B and D. A generally similar arrangement as was envisaged for the ruby laser—enclosing the active material between mirrors—was used by Javan and his co-workers, as shown in the schematic diagram of Fig. 9.4. After some adjustments to determine the best conditions—of gas composition and pressure and of current in the tube—laser action at the 1·15 μm infra-red line was achieved.

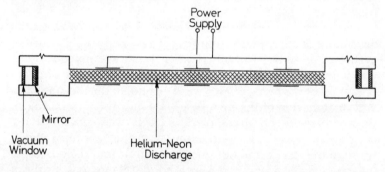

Fig. 9.4   Schematic of Javan's helium-neon laser. The ends of the tube are slightly flexible so that the mirrors can be adjusted to be accurately parallel.

There were two main characteristics of the gas laser which distinguished it from the ruby laser. In the first place, the gas laser worked continuously, giving a steady infra-red beam for as long as the current was passed. This is because the need for an enormously intense light flash, to produce the conditions for amplification, is absent in the gas laser. Secondly, the line given by the helium-neon laser was very much sharper than that of the ruby—so much so that it proved impossible to measure at first, and special techniques had to be developed in order to estimate the sharpness of the line. The reason for this is clear. The act of exposing the ruby crystal to an intense flash heats the crystal, which expands and changes the mirror separation, so changing the wavelength of the light given out. In the gas laser, a small, steady current flows through the gas, which soon reaches an even temperature, so that the wavelength of the laser radiation stays steady.

Soon after the development of the helium-neon infra-red laser, it was found possible to use the higher energy metastable helium atoms (Fig. 9.3) to produce excited neon, and thereby to make the laser give out visible (red) light. This was made possible by using a type of mirror which reflects some wavelengths better than others. Thus it is possible to make a mirror which reflects red light very strongly but which hardly reflects the infra-red radiation which the first laser emitted. When the red-reflecting mirrors are used, the infra-red radiation in the laser cannot build up sufficiently to make the laser work at this wavelength.

The arrival of the helium-neon laser led the way to the development of very large numbers of gas lasers, using a variety of gases. The vital spadework done by Javan and his co-workers was a masterpiece of systematic, painstaking study and the operation of the first gas laser was a tribute to the thoroughness and imagination of the investigators. Once the way had been shown, literally hundreds of new lasers were made, giving radiation at wavelengths stretching from the near ultra-violet, through the visible and out into the far infra-red regions of the spectrum. Indeed it almost appeared that if one took a tube of gas (any gas), placed it between suitable mirrors and passed an electric current through the gas, then one was almost certain to produce a laser. There were perhaps two rules in the event of failure, namely (1) make it bigger and (2) add helium. There are in fact many working lasers for which we know very little of the details of operation.

In many cases, the powers generated are very small. Among the more powerful sources of this kind are those using argon, krypton and carbon dioxide. Argon and krypton lasers are of interest in that they produce a number of intense lines in the visible spectrum—can indeed be arranged so that several colours appear together and give the sensation of white light (which is normally the result of the continuous red/orange/ yellow/green/blue/violet of the spectrum). The carbon dioxide laser produces an infra-red beam with a wavelength of 10·6 micrometres (0·00106 cm). The remarkable feature of this laser is the very high continuous power produced. At present, such systems can produce the same power continuously as the first ruby laser produced in its brief, thousandth-of-a-second flash. Such beams will, for example, burn holes in materials such as brick at an impressive rate—several centimetres per second.

Despite the remarkable intensity of the radiation produced by most solid and gas lasers (which arises from the extreme directionality of the beams produced), they are mostly very inefficient. The power given out by most of the continuously operating gas lasers is only a minute fraction of that put in. Thus for the helium-neon laser which produces a beam with a power of $\frac{1}{1000}$ watt, it is generally necessary to put in about 10–20 watts. Argon ion lasers are somewhat better, but even in these only about one-hundredth of the input power emerges in the laser beam. The reason for this is not hard to find. If we look at the spectrum of the light from, say, neon or argon atoms, we see an enormous number of lines—the energy of the emerging radiation is spread over very many lines, only one (or a very few) of which can produce a laser beam. When a discharge is struck in many gases, atoms become excited to a vast number of different states and can return to the unexcited state via a very large number of possible routes. Only few of these take in the laser line, so only a small fraction of the input power can emerge in the laser beam. The notable exception to the generally low efficiency of the gas laser is the carbon dioxide laser, which has the astonishingly high efficiency of 25%. As with the other gases, there is an enormous number of excited states of carbon dioxide, and many routes by which excited molecules can return to the normal state. However a very large number of the possible routes have to go via the observed 10·6 micrometre line, so that a high efficiency is possible in this case.

Quite apart from the inherent limitations referred to above, there may be other factors which limit the output power of a laser. In the case of helium-neon, the conditions for getting the necessary population inversion are met only when the current through the gas is kept to a fairly low value. If the current is made too large, the system ceases to work. In contrast, the argon ion laser works well at very large currents—in fact—the higher the better. However in this case the limit is set by the material of the tube containing the discharge. When a really fierce discharge is let loose in the tube, the inside walls of the tube are vaporised and the tube rapidly collapses. In this case, the big problem is of finding materials to withstand the rugged conditions imposed by the discharge. Early models employed quartz: more recently graphite and aluminium oxide have been tried with considerable improvements.

With solid lasers such as ruby or rare-earth-doped materials, there are two main problems. Since some of the energy of the excited atoms goes in heating the crystal, the efficiency is limited through this cause. The theoretical limit to the efficiency of a ruby laser is about 40%, depending on the kind of light source used for excitation. However in practice much lower efficiencies are obtained. In part, these are due to the presence of imperfections in the crystals used. There is considerable scope for improvement in this area. Crystal-growing at present owes as much to art as to science.

CHAPTER TEN

Semiconductors and the semiconductor laser

There is a third class of lasers in which a rather different method is used from those of the lasers discussed in the previous two chapters. The fundamental basis of operation is of course the same for all systems. In the semiconductor laser, however, a radically different method is used to produce the necessary inversion of population. Moreover, the occurrence of spontaneous and stimulated emission arises in a somewhat different manner from that in the systems discussed thus far.

A common characteristic of the gas and ruby-type lasers which have been considered in previous chapters is that the processes basic to the production of laser action can be thought of as happening in isolated atoms. This is easy to accept for gas lasers because in these devices the atoms are, on average, very far apart. Thus in the helium-neon mixture used for this laser, the average distance between atoms is about three hundred times the diameter of the atom. Since atoms do not affect one another appreciably unless they are very close indeed, we may take it that the atoms behave as though undisturbed. The situation is less simple in the case of ruby, for here we are dealing with a solid. The atoms surrounding the important chromium ion are very close indeed and would normally be expected to disturb the chromium so much that our simple picture of excitation and de-excitation by photons should not hold. If the chromium ion is being joggled by its neighbours, how can it send out light of such a constant frequency? The reason is that, when the chromium ion is excited by absorbing radiation, the electrons around the atom which are excited lie rather close to the nucleus—they are not, as in the case of neon atoms, on the outside of the atom. Thus although the chromium ion is subject to some jostling by its rather close neighbours, the inner electrons which take part in the laser emission are scarcely disturbed and the atom behaves in roughly the same way as it would if isolated.

The situation in a semiconductor is quite different. The atoms of the semiconductor are very close together, but the laser emission is *not* due to inner electrons. Before discussing how stimulated emission does occur in a semiconductor, it will be useful to examine the particular characteristics of this interesting (and in recent years technologically important) class of materials. This takes us into a lengthy digression on the properties and structure of these materials.

As the name implies, the (electrical) conductivity of semiconductors is not very high—as is the case for metals—nor is it very low, such as that of glass and other insulators. The main feature which distinguishes conduction in a semiconductor from that in a metal is the dependence of conductivity on temperature. Metals become poorer conductors as the temperature is increased. The conductivity of semiconductors increases with rising temperature. This suggests that there must be some rather basic difference in the mechanism of conduction in the two cases and this is indeed so.

Studies of the behaviour of metals lead us to the idea that when individual metal atoms come together to form a solid, one or two of the outermost electrons become detached. Consider, for example, the case of sodium. In the vapour of sodium, where the atoms are isolated from one another, the electrons occupy regions round the atom as indicated in Fig. 10.1. Note that there is one electron which is significantly farther from the nucleus than the rest. When atoms of sodium are brought together to form a solid, the outermost electron of each atom is so disturbed by the surrounding atoms that it appears to break loose. We thus have the situation shown in Fig. 10.2 in which there is a regular array of sodium *ions* (since each has lost an electron) and a "sea" of loose electrons which appear to be able to wander almost without let or hindrance through the crystal. Indeed it is

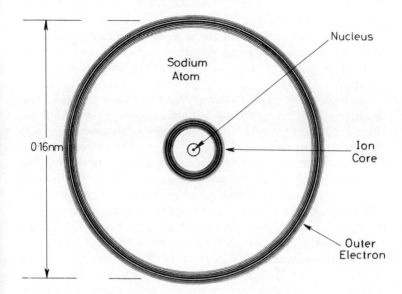

Fig. 10.1   Regions occupied by electrons round an isolated sodium atom.

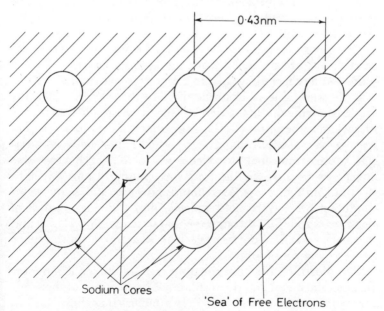

Fig. 10.2   The situation in metallic sodium.

for precisely this reason that sodium is a good conductor of electricity. If we apply a voltage to a piece of sodium (or indeed of any metal), there are vast numbers of electrons immediately ready to be swept through the metal—in other words to conduct electricity.

An important point to note is that the *number* of electrons floating around in the metal is fixed. For the case of sodium, there is just one for each atom. Only the outermost electron is shaken off—the rest cling tightly to the nucleus. Why then does the conductivity of a metal change at all with temperature? The conductivity of a material is a measure of how freely electrons can move through the metal. Although the electrons which provide the conduction are free in the sense of being detached from their parent atoms, they still have to push their way through the array of atoms (ions) forming the crystal. Thus they will not be able to streak unimpeded from one end of the sample to the other, but will collide with the metal ions *en route*. The reason why metals become poorer conductors as they become hotter is simply that, as the temperature rises, the metal ions wobble more from their normal positions. There is thus a greater chance that electrons will be scattered out of their path as they stream along the sample.

The opposite extreme to the metal is the insulator. In this case *no* electrons are detached from the atoms when they form a solid, so there is nothing to carry an electric current.

If we were able to examine directly the way in which the atoms of a semiconductor were arranged, we should find that in many cases, the tetrahedral arrangement of Fig. 10.3 was present. We should find that generally the region between adjacent atoms contained two electrons, so that each atom was linked, or bonded, to the four surrounding atoms by eight electrons, in four pairs. We should, however, unless the semiconductor were very cold indeed, find quite a number of electrons wandering through the material. We should also find that here and there only *one* electron was present in the space between adjacent atoms.

This illustrates the "intermediateness" of the semiconductor between the metal and the insulator. The electrons of the semiconductor atoms are not so loosely attached that they fly off as soon as the atoms are packed together. Nor are they so tightly

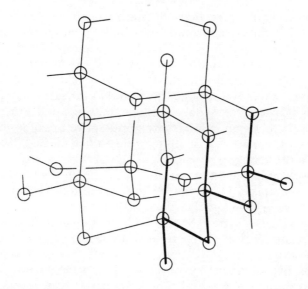

Fig. 10.3 Arrangement of atoms in certain semiconductor materials.

bound to the atom that they will not shake loose at all. At low temperatures, most of the electrons *are* sitting comfortably in their linking position. As the temperature is raised, the atoms vibrate more and electrons tend to be shaken off. Here, however, we see a crucial difference from a metal. The more we heat the semiconductor, the more electrons we shake off. In contrast to the metal, where the number of freed electrons does not change, the number in a semiconductor increases very rapidly as the material is heated. Thus for a typical semiconductor, the number of conducting electrons produced in this way will double for a rise in temperature of only a few degrees.

Germanium and silicon are two semiconductors which form structures such as are shown in Fig. 10.3. In the isolated state, each of these atoms has four outermost electrons. Thus the eight electrons required to form the four bonds around each atom can be obtained by the simple device of having adjacent atoms each contribute an electron to the link. It would seem that a similar structure could arise if we had equal numbers of two different atoms, provided the sum of the numbers of outer electrons added up to eight. Although reality turns out to be far more complicated than this simple picture suggests, there are in fact many semiconductors made of equal mixtures of atoms which have three and five outer electrons.

Let us look a little more closely into the way in which a semiconductor conducts electricity. Clearly the "shaken-off" electrons can move through the crystal in the same way as the electrons in a metal. What about the "missing link"—the place where the electron came from? Suppose we apply a voltage between the ends of a sample, as illustrated in Fig. 10.4. As shown, the voltage will tend to push electrons from right to left. An electron in the bond nearest to the "single-electron" bond can rather easily be persuaded to hop into the vacant place. This leaves a vacancy in *its* bond, so a further jump can occur, by the next electron to the right. This can go on until we have moved the "missing link" right through the crystal. The net result of this is that the electric charge has moved through the crystal, by the movement of the "hole" (as the missing link is called) through the crystal. Thus for a perfectly pure material, either of identical atoms (like germanium) or of exactly equal numbers of properly arranged atoms (like gallium arsenide), we expect conduction to occur by freed electrons moving one way through the crystal and holes moving in the opposite direction. Since the freeing of each electron leaves one hole behind, there will clearly be equal numbers of each in a crystal.

Early work on semiconductors proved extremely difficult to do because it was found that the conductivity of these materials

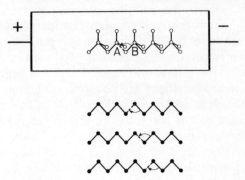

Fig. 10.4   Effect of applying a voltage to a semiconductor. Electron moves from completed bond (B) to bond with missing electron (A).

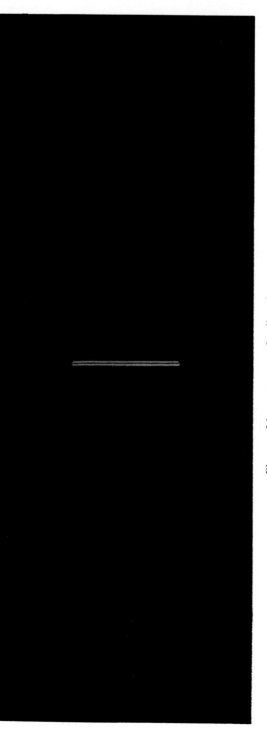

Plate 3 Line spectrum of sodium lamp.

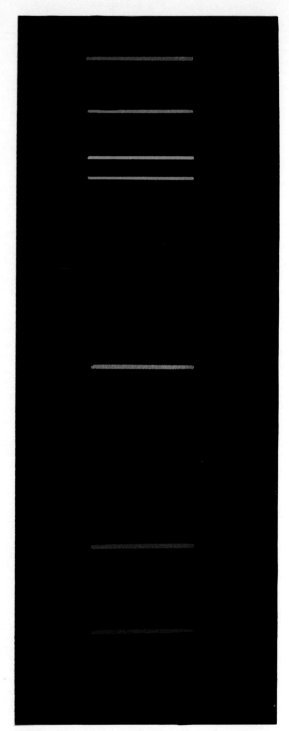

Plate 4 Line spectrum of helium lamp.

was extremely sensitive to purity. Minute traces—scarcely detectable amounts—of some kinds of impurity could make an enormous difference to the conducting properties. We can readily see why this should be. Suppose we introduce a small amount of an impurity which has *five* electrons round it into a semiconductor whose atoms normally have four. If the impurity atom sits in place of one of the normal atom, only four of its electrons are required to make bonds and the fifth is free to wander off through the crystal—and to take part in conduction. Or, suppose we put in an atom with only *three* outer electrons. When this intruder sits in the crystal, it will form one single-electron link with one of its neighbours—that is, it will provide a hole which, like a freed electron, can take part in conduction. Materials with an excess number of wandering electrons are described as "*n*-type". Those which have more holes than electrons are known as "*p*-type". The reason for the profound effect of minute amounts of impurity is that, except at high temperatures, the number of electrons (or holes) in a pure material is very small. At room temperature, we may have only one electron for every ten thousand million atoms of the pure material. So, if we have one impurity atom for every hundred million normal atoms, there will be a hundred times as many electrons (or holes) from the impurities as from the normal atoms.

What happens if one of the wandering electrons (not the "hopping", bond-to-bond, ones) finds itself near to a hole? It will clearly be sorely tempted to abandon its nomadic existence and jump into place between the two atoms concerned. Now the mere fact that the loose electron *was* loose means that it has more energy when wandering about the crystal than it has when lying comfortably in place between the atoms. (We had, after all, to shake it out of place to get it loose—had, in fact, to give it some energy to free it.) The change from the wandering state to the "fixed" one means that some excess energy has to be disposed of, just as was so for the chromium ion in ruby or the excited atom in a gas. The excess energy emerges as radiation, just as it may for the other materials mentioned. Now we see the possibilities of a laser in the offing. Since radiation is emitted when the electron and hole recombine, we should expect that *stimulated* emission could occur. If our wandering electron hovers near a hole when a quantum of the right energy comes along, it may be pushed into place, to the accompaniment of stimulated emission. We thus see the semi-conductor counterpart of de-excitation of excited atoms in a gas.

In the same way that lower-state gas atoms can absorb a quantum, so the semiconductor can absorb. This happens when the radiation quantum dislodges an electron and sets it free to wander through the crystal. As in the case of a gas or other type of laser system, we shall get a net amplification if there is an excess of electrons in the more energetic (i.e. wandering) state over the number of holes into which they may fall.

If a piece of n-type semiconductor is intimately joined to some p-type and if a current is passed across the junction, we can in some circumstances create the necessary population inversion. (In practice, we use a single piece of crystal and place the right impurities in contact with the surface: on heating the crystal, the impurities go part of the way into the crystal and so create the necessary junction between n- and p-type inside the crystal.) A typical form of crystal for a semiconductor laser is shown in Fig. 10.5. We have no need for external mirrors because the surfaces of these materials are quite good reflectors. Thus the surfaces of the crystal (Fig. 10.5) serve as mirrors and so make laser action possible. Gallium arsenide is one successful laser material, as is also the phosphide. The wavelength emitted by gallium arsenide is 0·84 micrometres—just into the infra-red region. Gallium phosphide gives a wavelength of 0·64 micrometres. A useful and rather unusual feature of these lasers is that by making a crystal containing both arsenic and phosphorus, the wavelength of the laser radiation emitted can be adjusted

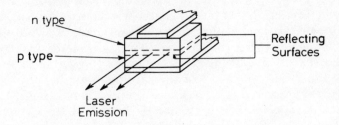

Fig. 10.5   Form of typical semiconductor laser. (No mirrors are needed. The faces of the crystal serve as reflectors.)

between the limits given above. This is in contrast to the behaviour of the other solid lasers discussed above and to that of gas lasers. In these cases it is not possible to adjust the wavelength of the laser emission, except by a minute amount.

In general, the current needed to make a semiconductor laser work is rather large, so that we have a heating problem, as in the case of the ruby laser. It is usual therefore to use short pulses of current which may, however, follow one another quite rapidly. Thus a typical gallium arsenide laser may produce tens of thousands of pulses per second.

Semiconductor lasers have interesting possibilities in the field of communications and we shall refer to them again in Chapter 13.

CHAPTER ELEVEN

Trends in laser development

As mentioned in Chapter 9, lasers have been made to work over a very wide range of wavelengths, from the ultra-violet to the far infra-red. By and large, the wavelength which a laser produces is governed by the kind of atom or molecule which is used. In the same way that a sodium lamp always gives the same yellow light—the result of the way in which the sodium atom is built—so lasers give a wavelength which depends on the characteristics of the atoms taking part. This would seem therefore to impose a severe restriction—we can on the face of it produce a laser beam of a particular wavelength only if there exists in nature an atom which itself emits at that wavelength. (The restriction is in fact more severe than this: we must be able to produce the population inversion needed.)

In fact, there exists a number of ways in which a variety of additional lasers and laser-type sources may be made. One of these was discovered by accident when, in an experiment designed to produce very intense laser pulses, a glass cell containing nitrobenzene was placed between a ruby laser rod and one of the mirrors, as shown in Fig. 11.1. (In this case a separate mirror was used instead of putting the mirror coating on the end of the ruby.) When the ruby laser was operated, it was found that in addition to the normal ruby light, light of other colours emerged from the end of the laser. This arose from an effect with which physicists and chemists had been familiar for over half a century, known as the Raman effect. When a light from a

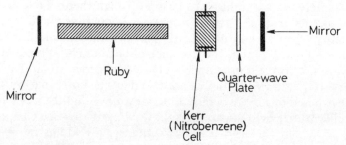

Fig. 11.1 Arrangement which led to the accidental discovery of the Raman laser. The Kerr cell and quarter-wave plate are for Q-spoiling; (see p. 96).

source giving an intense sharp spectral line, such as a mercury lamp, was directed at certain kinds of molecule, tiny amounts of light emerged with a wavelength slightly different from that of the light going in. Some of the energy of the ingoing light quantum is taken up by the molecule and serves to make the atoms in the molecule vibrate faster than usual. The light which is scattered out of the molecule thus has a slightly smaller energy and hence a longer wavelength than that of the illuminating beam. Normally this effect is very small and the "Raman-scattered" light is extremely weak. When however a laser is used as a source, the intensity is so high that quite large intensities of Raman-scattered light can be produced. When the Raman scattering material is between the laser mirrors, then the light travelling along the axis can build up intensity in the same way that the laser light does. Now the amount by which Raman-shifted lines differ in wavelength from the exciting line depends on the type of molecule. Thus by choosing the appropriate material to put in the Raman cell in this kind of laser, a large selection of new laser frequencies becomes possible. They are, however, necessarily at fixed wavelengths—the laser frequency cannot be continuously tuned in this arrangement.

There is another way in which lasers may be used to produce intense beams of light with wavelengths which might otherwise not be available, which, as in the Raman system mentioned above, depends on the very high intensity generated by the laser. In this, the laser can produce light whose wavelength is one half of that given by the laser itself. The effect arises from the behaviour of atoms in certain types of crystal when an

extremely intense light wave passes through them. To borrow
an analogy from the acoustic field, we know that the differing
quality of sound emitted by different instruments playing the
same note arises from the presence of harmonics. We are also
aware that certain instruments give a purer tone when played
very softly than when blown hard. When the atoms in a crystal
are exposed to a beam of radiation, they move slightly to and fro
as the electric field due to the light wave oscillates (see Chapter
2). Provided the field is not too intense, the atoms move in
sympathy with the incoming light and can be thought of as
minute antennae, broadcasting at exactly the same frequency as
that at which they are made to oscillate. We could in fact think
of the light which passes out of the crystal as being due to the
combined antenna action of the atoms in the crystal.

If the intensity of the incoming beam is very large, the movement of the atoms does not exactly follow the field of the wave.
In the same way that the musical instrument generates harmonics when blown hard, so the motion of the atoms in the
crystal generate harmonics of the incoming wave. Thus if an
intense pulse of (infra-red) radiation from a neodymium glass
laser is sent into a crystal of ammonium dihydrogen phosphate,
a brilliant flash of green light emerges from the crystal. The
wavelength of the neodymium radiation is 1·06 micrometres
and that of the "second harmonic" emission is 0.53 micrometres—in the green part of the spectrum. If the red light from
a ruby laser is used a beam of ultra-violet radiation is produced.
It proves possible to convert a large fraction of the power of a
laser beam into its second harmonic—and in fact to repeat the
process with the second harmonic so generated. If the green
light from the neodymium laser-plus-phosphate crystal is
passed into a second crystal ultraviolet radiation of wavelength
$\frac{0·53}{2} = 0·265$ micrometres can be produced. There is a limit to
the extent to which this can be done. Although in principle we
should be able to carry the process a stage further, this can be
done only if we have the right kind of crystal which will not
absorb the harmonic radiation. In the case of the example
given above, there is no suitable crystal known which does not
absorb radiation of wavelength 0·132 micrometres. (Crystals
which are transparent to ultra-violet radiation of this wave-

length do exist but they do not have the type of structure needed for harmonic generation to be possible.)

Although as mentioned above we generally have no control over the wavelength which atoms emit, there is a tantalising possibility which arises in connection with certain organic materials, known as chelates. These are large molecules, containing many atoms in the form of three-dimensional frameworks and it is possible to build into such structures atoms of the type suitable for laser action, especially those of the rare earth series (see Table 8.1). It is found that the wavelength emitted by rare earth atoms in molecules of this type does in fact depend somewhat on the configuration of the molecule. We have a certain amount of control over the structure of such molecules and we can tack on different groups of molecules in various places. If, then, molecules of this type can be persuaded to act as laser materials, there appears the possibility of adjusting the wavelength emitted by suitable manipulation of the surrounding molecular architecture.

Laser action has in fact been obtained in a number of chelate molecules, generally in solution. Excitation of the atoms in the molecule is by exposure to a light flash, as in the case of ruby and crystal lasers. Two problems arise with these materials. In the first place, they are not very transparent to the light required for excitation, so that one tends only to excite the laser atoms on the surface of the sample. Secondly, there is a tendency for the molecule to be broken up by the radiation at the high intensities required. At this time, the prospects for high-power, versatile chelate lasers seem not too favourable, although progress is being made and the scope for further development is by no means exhausted.

In the direction of producing higher and higher powers from lasers of the ruby type, an ingenious technique known as "Q-spoiling" is adopted. If we examine the intense red flash from a ruby laser of the type described in Chapter 8 we find that the light does not come out in a single flash, but rather as a whole succession of extremely brief ones. This happens simply because as soon as we have produced enough excited atoms in the crystal to cause the laser to operate stimulated emission occurs and the atoms are de-excited. If the light from the flash tube is still illuminating the ruby, then a further supply of excited atoms is

produced, but again as soon as enough are present another laser
flash occurs. This goes on for as long as the light from the flash
tube is on—typically about a thousandth of a second. It would
clearly be an advantage if we could prevent laser action from
starting until we had produced a really large number of excited
atoms. Then if we could "switch on" the laser, we should get
one truly enormous flash. This is not difficult to arrange if we
put one of the ruby laser mirrors a little way from the end of the
ruby, instead of coating the ruby with a mirror surface. If we
then put a rotating sectored wheel, as shown in Fig. 11.2, between
the ruby and the mirror, we can arrange that the illuminating
flash occurs while a solid part of the wheel is in the way. Since
no reflection can occur at the mirror, we do not get the necessary
high intensity of light in the ruby and so laser action cannot
start. As soon as a gap in the wheel moves into the path to the
mirror, reflection at the mirror occurs and the laser then
operates, rapidly releasing an enormous amount of energy from
the large number of excited atoms present. There are a number
of other ways of achieving the same result. Thus we may use a
Kerr cell (Chapter 4), applying a voltage in such a way that the
laser can operate for only a very brief period. The details need
not concern us. Suffice it to say that when this method is used,
the laser produces a very large amount of energy in a single,
very short pulse—lasting perhaps only a fraction of a millionth
of a second, but producing an intensity far far higher than that
ever produced by any ordinary source of light. The intensities

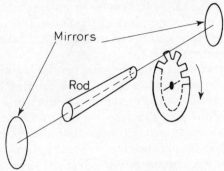

Fig. 11.2   One of the ways of producing Q-spoiled pulses from a laser. The
tooth in the way of the beam prevents laser action starting until a large concentration of excited atoms in the ruby has been produced.

attainable are so high that a whole new field of physics of high-intensity radiation has become possible, together with a number of interesting technological possibilities, to which we return in Chapter 13.

In the operation of a high-power solid state laser, such as ruby or neodymium in glass, the output generally consists of a large number of waves of slightly different frequencies. This arises because there are many ways, with a cavity which is very much longer than the wavelength of the light, in which waves can reflect back and forth in the manner required to produce laser action. Thus for waves passing back and forth along the axis of the laser, it is merely necessary that a whole-number of wavelengths will fit into the space between the mirrors. For a cavity 20 cm long, 200,000 waves of length 0·0001 cm will fit in. Equally, 199,999 waves of fractionally larger length will go. Since, in lasers of this type, the radiation available to start laser action spans a finite band of wavelengths, many such resonances are possible.

In many situations, the different modes of oscillation operate independently of one another, being described as "free-running". Depending precisely on what is happening in the laser, modes may come and go, or their frequencies may drift as, e.g., the length of the laser rod increases through expansion as a result of heating. In some circumstances, however, the phases of the many modes may become locked together. This can occur if, e.g., a layer of a suitable bleachable dye is inserted in the beam within the laser cavity. The effect of locking the phases of the laser modes ("phase-locking" or "mode-locking") is dramatic. If we imagine a large number of wavetrains with slightly different frequencies all superposed with random phases, the result (Fig. 11.3) is a long train with irregular amplitude. If, however, the phases of the modes are all locked together, the resultant of combining the modes is an extremely short-duration pulse. In the neighbourhood of the pulse, the modes combine to give a large resultant; in all other parts of the wavetrain, the waves tend to cancel and produce a small resultant. By this method, pulses of incredible sharpness—of duration much less than a million millionth of a second can be produced.

The inevitable problem arose, when the possibility of producing such short pulses was considered, of how one would be

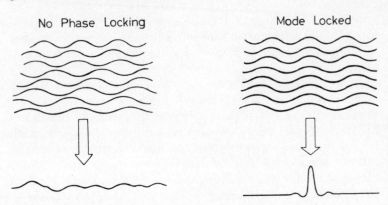

Fig. 11.3(a)   Combination of many trains of waves with random phases. The result is a small, irregular disturbance.
Fig. 11.3(b)   When the waves are locked in step, a very intense, short pulse is produced.

able to measure such short time intervals. Conventionally, the most sensitive methods available for measuring such short intervals involve displaying the signal on a cathode ray tube, on which a horizontal sweep indicates time as a co-ordinate measured across the face of the tube. Unfortunately, the fastest electronic circuitry at present available can produce a spot which sweeps across the face of the C.R. tube in about 10^{-10}–10^{-9} sec. Thus an event lasting only about 10^{-12} sec would be barely detected in a beam which ambled across the face of the tube in a leisurely ten thousand millionth of a second. A totally different method is in fact used for these measurements. This is a method which relies on the fact that, in some circumstances, fluorescence may be produced in certain materials by the absorption of two photons simultaneously. In the normal way, materials may absorb an incident quantum and become excited. Return to the ground state may occur either directly or via intermediate levels. In some situations, the energy required to produce excitation may be just double that of the incident photons. Now, normally, the chance of two photons arriving sufficiently nearly simultaneously at an atom to cause excitation is extremely small. If, however, the intensity of the incident wave is high enough, there is a good chance of excitation through the simultaneous absorption of *two* photons. If the excited atoms return directly to the ground state, emitting one photon, radiation will be emitted with a wavelength one half of that of the exciting photon. Thus if a Nd in glass laser is used, emitting infra-red radiation of wavelength 1·064 µm, the fluorescence emitted through two-photon absorption will have a wavelength of 0·53 µm—in the middle of the visible spectrum. If, then, a beam of radiation consisting of a train of light pulses of duration 10^{-12} sec is reflected at a mirror so that forward and backward trains of waves pass through a suitable fluorescing medium, fluorescence will be observed at high intensity where the forward and backward pulses overlap. Since the velocity of light in a typical fluorescing medium is about 2×10^8 m/sec, the length of a 10^{-12} sec pulse is 0·2 mm. Thus a burst of light from a region 0·2 mm long will be observed (Fig. 11.4) and measurement of the length of this pulse gives the duration of the light pulse.

The high power of a laser is by no means its only important feature. The fact that the laser gives a *coherent* beam of light (see Chapter 1) gives it a whole range of potentialities, in the fields of

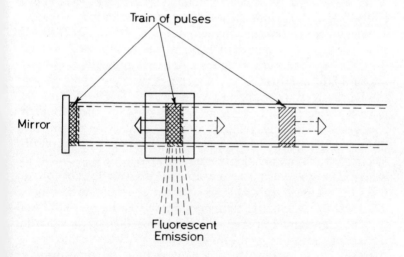

Fig. 11.4 How the duration of ultra-short pulses is measured. Pulses travelling in opposite directions overlap in a fluorescent cell. Light emerges from this region: by measuring the length of this region, the duration of the pulse is determined.

measurement and communication. For many of these applications, it is essential that the wavelength of the emission remain constant to a very high degree. (In the case of radio waves used for broadcasting, any wandering of the wavelength of the carrier wave would mean that the receiving set had constantly to be re-tuned. The same considerations apply to a laser used for this purpose.) Although, as mentioned in Chapter 9, the gas laser produces a much steadier wavelength than, e.g., the ruby laser, the wavelength does nevertheless wander by more than can be tolerated for many purposes. The problem is that although the wavelength of the light given out depends on the atom, it also depends on the speed with which the atom moves—for the same reason that the sound of a train hooter changes as the train passes us. Since in a gas (and even in a solid) the atoms are not stationary, the wavelength of the light received from them covers a range of values. Now the precise wavelength which a laser emits depends mainly on the distance between the laser mirrors. A high intensity builds up, by multiple reflections, only if the mirror separation is a whole number of wavelengths. Thus if the length of the laser changes, so does the wavelength emitted. Anything that causes the length of the laser to change —mechanical vibration, or changes in temperature—will cause the laser wavelength to wander. It is possible to overcome this tendency in a number of ways. One method entails mounting one of the mirrors on a piezo-electric crystal, whose thickness can be changed by applying a voltage to it. The light from the laser is collected on a detector which gives an output which changes if the laser wavelength varies. The varying output can be used to generate a voltage which, when applied to the piezo-electric crystal, causes the mirror to move in such a way as to keep the laser wavelength constant. In this way it is possible to keep the wavelength stable to within extremely small limits. Thus stabilities of better than one part in ten thousand million may be maintained in this way, so making the laser a suitable device for radio-like communication.

In the early days of lasers, costs were high, partly reflecting ing the high cost of developing the necessary technologies. Moreover they often required some skill in adjustment and were difficult to maintain. Since then considerable advances have been made so that the present generation of lasers makes little demand on the experimenters' skills. Although the cost is still high compared, e.g., with that of other types of source, the stage is approaching where these devices become consumable, plug-in components like the ordinary electric light bulb.

Can we give any indication of the likely or desirable trends in the development of lasers of the future? So far as existing types of laser are concerned, there will clearly be efforts to improve the rather low efficiency of most laser systems. It seems improbable that any dramatic new developments will arise in gas lasers employing monatomic gases since most of these have by now been examined. There may be scope for lasers using molecular gases although here again most of the common ones have been tried. In some ways it seems strange that, of all the molecular gases used so far, carbon dioxide alone yields a laser with a respectably high efficiency. One interesting point about the CO_2 laser centres on the possibility of making a laser operate efficiently by using excited CO_2 molecules produced chemically, for example by burning oil. When CO_2 is produced in this way, the resultant gas certainly contains molecules in excited states. In fact, laser action has been produced in this way, but only at extremely low efficiency. An efficient laser of this type would be of interest in that its operation would be independent of the provision of electrical power to sustain the discharge. Even in its present form, the CO_2 laser is likely to be the subject of further study, since its continuous power capability and its high efficiency make it a possible tool in many engineering and technological applications. Some of these are discussed in Chapter 13.

Development of lasers giving visible light will probably be heavily influenced by their applicability in colour-display situations—for example in future forms of television or colour projection systems. The question here would seem to be whether gas lasers, of the kinds described in Chapter 9 or solid state lasers employing Raman or harmonic generation effects are likely to provide the more effective tools. The present progress in solid state lasers running continuously and being operated by ordinary filament lamps augurs well for a system of long life, in which the only replacement needed would be the lamp. The laser rod/mirror part would have virtually unlimited life. The gas laser would appear to be less satisfactory in that the life would be limited by the filament within the system, which cannot easily be replaced, or by the fact that eventually the gas in the tube gets absorbed on the walls. From some points of view, the semiconductor laser offers great potential inasmuch as it can be made small and is simple in operation. The present range of these devices is somewhat limited, but there remain a wide variety of possible materials to be examined.

CHAPTER TWELVE

Similarities and differences—
laser light and ordinary light

Thus far we have stressed two features of laser light sources which distinguish them from ordinary sources. They are *directional* and the radiation which they produce is *coherent*. The directional characteristic is seen to emerge from the fact that lasers require mirrors to enable a large intensity to build up. This can happen only for a rather well-defined direction. The coherent property serves to tell us that when a radiation field stimulates excited atoms to emit, the emitted radiation is in step with that producing the de-excitation. We cannot, however, say quite simply that laser radiation is coherent whereas that of other sources is not, since radiation may show a greater or lesser degree of coherence. We shall discuss below in some detail the significance of coherence and shall answer the question "is there any intrinsic difference between laser light and ordinary light?" The question may have more than academic interest. Man's inherent curiosity leads him to wonder whether civilisations similar to our own are to be found in other regions of the universe. (Statistically, the chances of such civilisations existing within range of our own are high. Thus there are about 10^{11} stars in our own galaxy and a corresponding number of galaxies. Not only is it likely that other civilisations exist—it is possible that at this moment, someone, somewhere is reading a book on lasers!) If such civilisations exist and their inhabitants share our curiosity one can expect that efforts will be made to communicate. How might one do this? If we assume a comparable level of development on the part of our cosmic neighbours, we can assume that they will be able to construct masers or lasers. Possession of such a device greatly increases the chances of communication being possible because the laser is able to radiate large powers along relatively narrow beams. One watt of power from a laser which radiates into a conical beam one twentieth of a degree wide is equivalent, for the distant observer, to an "ordinary" source of about ten million watts. We could assume that our neighbours would, in attempts to communicate, direct a maser or laser beam at us and, by some suitable coding, try to transmit information to us. If we receive such a beam, would we know that it came from a laser? If we observed a strong neon line at 0·633 micrometres (the red laser wavelength) in the light from a distant region, could we distinguish this from the same line emitted by a mass of hot gas? We should be suspicious if this were the *only* neon line seen, for we should expect to get many more if we had simply an incandescent mass of neon. However, is there any measurable difference between the light from a laser and that from an ordinary source?

The notion of coherence can be discussed in connection with the effects of interference exhibited by light waves. Plate 2 shows the interference pattern (Newton's Rings) obtained when light of a single wavelength is reflected at the surfaces of a lens and a flat plate, placed close together. The occurrence of such rings is easily understood in terms of the wave picture of a light beam. In some places, the waves from the two surfaces leave in step and give a bright ring. In others, the waves are out of step and their effects cancel, so a dark ring appears. Suppose that the lens is placed at a long distance from the flat. Should we still expect to observe Newton's Rings? In practice, if we use a sodium or mercury lamp, we do *not* observe the rings unless the surfaces are fairly close together. In view of our discussions in Chapter 5 of the nature of light from an ordinary source, we are not surprised at this result. The source does *not* give out a coherent wave: the electromagnetic disturbance does *not* rise and fall rhythmically over long distances, because it is the result of emission by enormous numbers of atoms which are (spontaneously) emitting quite independently of one another. One classic experiment—the Michelson Interferometer—further

illustrates the way in which the limited coherence of an ordinary light source influences the interference effects which can be
produced. This instrument, shown in Fig. 12.1, consists of a
half-silvered plate and two fully-reflecting mirrors so arranged
that light from the left of the figure is divided at the plate so that
part continues to M_1 and part travels to M_2. After reflection
part of the light from M_2 goes through the plate and part of that

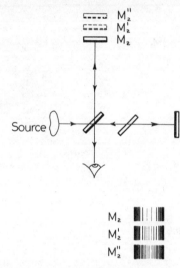

Fig. 12.1   The Michelson Interferometer.

from M_1 is reflected so that the two parts emerge together
towards the eye at the bottom of the diagram. If the mirrors are
not quite at right angles to one another, then straight-line
fringes are seen. As in the case of Newton's Rings, there are
some places where the two waves are in step and others where
they are out of step. Now if one of the mirrors is moved away
from its initial position (in which both mirrors are equidistant
from the plate) it is found that the fringes become less distinct
until eventually no fringes can be seen. In some cases a more
complicated behaviour ensues—with sodium light the fringes
become less distinct, then become clear again, then less distinct
again, cyclically for a range of movement. This arises because
the sodium lamp gives not one yellow line but two which are
close together. Nevertheless, quite apart from this complication,

we eventually reach a stage where no fringes can be observed. We can see how this could arise if we imagined the light given by the source to consist not of a truly continuous wave but as a whole sequence of sections of wave such as is shown in Fig. 12.2.

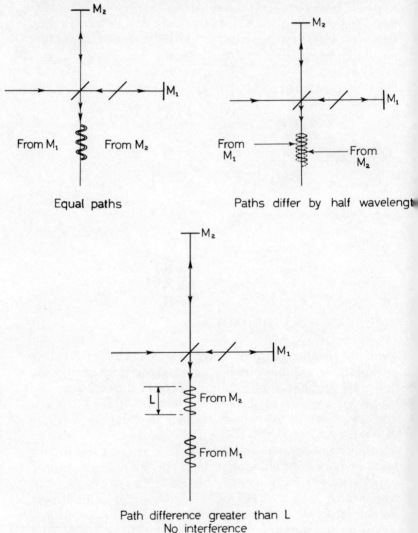

Fig. 12.2 Fringe formation in the Michelson Interferometer.

If the interferometer mirrors are at the same distance from the plates the waves travel equal distances from source to eye and so can overlap completely. If the paths followed are *exactly* equal then the waves reinforce and a bright fringe is seen. If the distances travelled differ by a half-wavelength (or, generally, an odd number of half-wavelengths) then the waves cancel and no light is seen. When one of the mirrors is moved, we can see that we shall eventually reach the stage where the two trains of waves do not overlap at all, so that they cannot interfere. We have shown a train of waves imagined to have been emitted for a very brief period. In fact the source is emitting all the time. By the time the wavetrain in Fig. 12.2(c) has taken the longer path to mirror M_2 and is emerging from the interferometer, it will be joined by waves emitted from the source at a later time. Why then do we not observe interference between these two waves? The answer is that we might be able to if we were able to make an almost instantaneous observation. However, the light which was emitted later came from a different collection of atoms which had forgotten how the early wavetrain was emitted. Thus the later waves may arrive in step or out of step with the early ones. Imagine this going on not with just two groups of waves but with many. Each pair of waves will give fringes, but the fringes will not all appear at the same place. If we add up the light from a large number of fringe patterns which, instead of neatly superposing, fall in random positions, we end up with uniform illumination—i.e. no fringes. We are led to a crude idea of a "coherence length" associated with the light beam. If two parts of the same beam are sent along paths of different length, then they will not interfere if the difference in their paths exceeds a certain distance—the coherence length.

Why is it that the radiation spontaneously emitted by atoms displays a finite coherence length? The result of the experiment with the Michelson interferometer shows that this is the case. There is another way of looking at the way radiation behaves which gives a useful insight into this property of radiation fields. We have already pointed out that a strictly monochromatic wave is one whose electric field (or any other oscillating property) rises and falls at exactly regular intervals. This implies that the wave is infinitely long and lasts for ever. In practice, we observe radiation from an atom for only a very

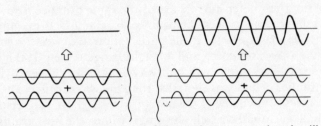

Fig. 12.3 For a time, two waves of almost the same wavelength will combine to give large oscillations. At a later time, however, the two waves would have got out of step and would tend to cancel.

brief period after it starts to return from the excited to the normal state—so the wave emitted by the atom certainly does *not* last for ever. Suppose now we had two truly infinite waves but with frequencies which differed very slightly from one another. If we sat and watched these waves go by, we should find that for a time they rose and fell almost in step (Fig. 12.3) and almost behaved as a single wave. After a time, however, the waves would—because they had slightly different wavelengths —get out of step, so that we would hardly detect anything. Later still they would be in step again and we would "see" them again. This is in fact what we observed in the case of the Michelson interferometer with a sodium lamp. Because two yellow lines

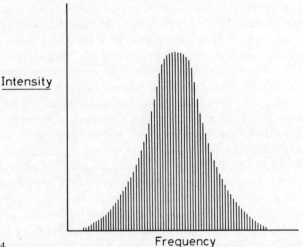

Fig. 12.4

are given out by such a lamp, there are positions of the Michelson mirror which make the two wavelengths emerge in step, so that we get fringes. For other mirror positions they emerge out of step. Imagine now not two but several frequencies all grouped round a particular value, as indicated in Fig. 12.4. If we add up the effect of such a collection of frequencies, we find that the result is a region over which the waves reinforce, to give a train of waves rather like that of Fig. 12.3 but that *everywhere* elsewhere, they tend to cancel and produce no effect. Thus we can conclude from this that the experiment with the Michelson interferometer shows that we must think of the atom as emitting the equivalent of a group of waves, with wavelengths spreading over a finite range. The way in which the energy is distributed over the different wavelengths is shown in Fig. 12.5 and is

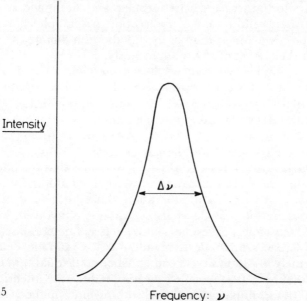

Intensity

$\Delta \nu$

Fig. 12.5   Frequency: ν

termed the *natural linewidth*. This is quite independent of any effects due to movement of the atoms during the emission—in fact it assumes that they are stationary. If they are moving, then the observed linewidth may well be much larger than the $\Delta \nu$ indicated above. Even when there are no effects due to motion (Doppler effects), atoms behave as though they give not a strictly monochromatic wave, but a group of waves whose frequencies cover a finite band. If we assemble a collection of truly monochromatic waves to form a group such as that described above, so that they reinforce one another and produce a limited train of waves, then we find that the time $\Delta\tau$ which the train takes to pass us is equal to $1/\Delta\upsilon$. Since the waves travel with the velocity c of light, the length of the train (corresponding to our notion of coherence length, discussed above) is $c \times \Delta\tau$. $\Delta\tau$ is called the "coherence time".

This, then, is the characteristic of non-laser light. If we examine the light from a large volume of emitting atoms, we find that it behaves as though it consisted of a superposition of vast numbers of wavetrains, each one corresponding to an emission from an individual atom. The wavetrains all have the same frequency (or rather band of frequencies) and the individual wavetrains arrive at the point of observation in a completely random fashion—a manifestation of the isolationism among the atoms when they are emitting spontaneously.

What kind of view may we take of laser light? The characteristics by which we can distinguish it from ordinary light are

1 that it is produced not by spontaneous emission, but by stimulated de-excitation of an atom by radiation, and

2 that it appears to be far more monochromatic than ordinary light from the same source.

The fact that a laser works at all indicates that the phases of the stimulated emission from an assembly of atoms are related to that of the stimulating radiation. Since in the case of spontaneous emission, no de-exciting radiation is involved, we may intuitively expect differences between laser and non-laser light.

Differences are indeed manifest if we examine beams of extremely low intensity. A consequence of the quantum nature of radiation is that when we steadily reduce the intensity of a beam (for example by putting absorbing filters in the beam) we reach the stage where we detect a succession of individual photons, rather than a continuous stream of energy. In the photocathode of whatever detector is used, the radiation *either* gives up an energy $h\upsilon$ to release an electron, which we then detect, *or* it does nothing. We find, however, that even from what we regard as a beam of constant intensity the arrival of photons does not occur at perfectly regular intervals. It is in the

way in which the photons arrive that differences between laser
and non-laser light may be observed.

Since the rate of arrival of photons fluctuates, we describe the
process in terms of probabilities. If we consider first non-laser
light, we find that for light of average intensity $\bar{I}$, the probability that at a given instant the intensity lies between I and
$I + dI$ is given by

$$p(I)\, dI \;=\; \frac{1}{\bar{I}} \exp\left(-I/\bar{I}\right) dI$$

If we set up an experiment to count photons over successive,
equal intervals of time, T, we may express the above result in
terms of the actual number n of photons arriving in the interval
and the mean number $\bar{n}$, which is given by $\bar{n}\,T \;=\; \bar{I}$. The resulting probability $p(n)$ that n photons arrive in time T is given by

$$p(n) \;=\; (1+\bar{n})^{-1}(1+\bar{n}^{-1})^{-n}$$

The form of the relation between $p(n, T)$ and n is given in Fig.
12.6. When the light from a thermal (non-laser) source is
studied in this way, the variation of p with n is indeed found to
follow the relation given above.

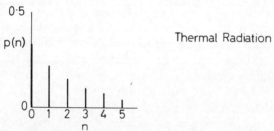

Fig. 12.6   Probability distribution for the arrival of photons from a thermal
light source ($\bar{n} = 2$).

With laser light, a quite different behaviour is expected. The
value of $p(n)$ is found to correspond closely to a Poisson distribution

$$p(n) \;=\; \frac{\bar{n}^{n} \exp\left(-\bar{n}\right)}{n!}$$

which is characteristic of a highly stable oscillator, in which the
amplitude is stabilised to its average value. As will be seen from

Figs. 12.7 and 12.6, the difference between the distributions is easily detected. Precautions are, however, necessary to avoid spurious instabilities in the laser experiment, which may arise from, e.g., fluctuations in the current in the tube.

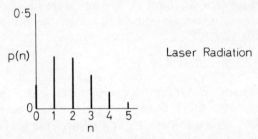

Fig. 12.7   Probability distribution for the arrival of photons from a laser source. ($\bar{n} = 2$).

Returning briefly to the space-communication aspect of the statistics of photons, let us speculate on the prospects of communication with the nearest star in our own galaxy—Alpha Centauri, which is at a distance of 0·65 parsecs (4×10^{13} km). If we assume that our neighbours have a 10,000 watt laser and mount this on a telescope, they should be able to direct the beam into a cone with an angle of one ten thousandth of a radian. If in turn we use the Mount Palomar 200 in. telescope to collect the beam, we should receive several photons per minute. It would be relatively easy, in a quite short time, to verify whether the photon statistics were those of thermal or of laser light (although there may be some difficulties due to atmospheric turbulence and scattering, necessitating the use of an orbiting telescope).

The mere verification or otherwise that the light from our neighbour is from a laser conveys rather little information—except by inference that intelligent beings are likely to be at the end of it. However one would next look for overall modulation effects, by which information could be transmitted.

The prospects for making contact with more distant parts of our own galaxy are somewhat feebler. From the furthest reaches, we may expect, from a similar laser transmitter, only one photon every sixty years, so that a rather considerable time would be involved in assessing the type of source, and of passing information. From the nature of the problem (due to the enormous scale of the universe) there is no need for impatience at the thought that a long time will be needed to decipher messages, since the transit time of the signal is not inconsiderable. Thus even from the other side of our own galaxy—from our cosmic next-door neighbours—the round-trip time for passing messages is about 200,000 years. We could afford, therefore, to spend a few generations' time in analysing the statistics of arriving photons to decipher our neighbours' news bulletins.

To return to earth and continue the discussion of the characteristics of laser light, we may mention certain features which derive from the way in which laser radiation is produced. As we have seen, the frequency of the light from an ordinary source covers a finite width, due either to the natural lifetime of the emitting atoms or to atomic motion, which gives rise to Doppler effects. Such linewidths may be observed by optical instruments of suitably high resolving power and have a shape as shown in Fig. 12.5. The corresponding pattern from light from a typical laser is as shown in Fig. 12.8. The spectrum in this

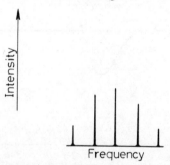

Fig. 12.8   Lasers may emit several extremely sharp lines at slightly different frequencies.

case consists of several extremely sharp lines—far sharper than those from an ordinary discharge of the same gas—with well-defined and constant separations. These arise from the way in which the radiation can resonate in the optical cavity. In Chapter 8 we described the way in which the intensity built up by referring to radiation travelling backwards and forwards between the mirrors, exactly along the axis. We were tacitly implying that the amplitude of the wave over the cross-section of the beam was constant and also that the wavelength was determined by the distance between the mirrors. This is a slightly over-simplified view of the situation. In practice, we find that there are many possible ways in which radiation may go back and forth. In one mode, the amplitude distribution is as shown in Fig. 12.9(a), with a maximum value on the axis and low values at the edges. For this mode, the wavelength is given by the condition that an exact number of half-wavelengths must fit into the space between the mirrors. In other modes, the distributions are as shown in Fig. 12.9(b) and (c). In these cases, the wavelengths differ very slightly from one another, so

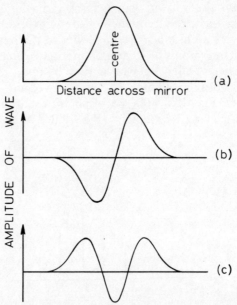

Fig. 12.9 Amplitude distribution across the beam in the three lowest-order modes. (a) (1, 0) mode; (b) (2, 0); (c) (3, 0).

that the output from the laser contains several frequencies. The intensity distributions are shown in Figs. 12.10 and 12.11. The presence of such modes is easily seen if the far-field diffraction pattern of the beam is examined. Typical mode patterns are shown in Fig. 12.12. Generally, the higher the power at which the laser is operated the larger the number of different modes

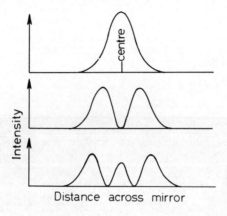

Fig. 12.10   Intensity distributions in the modes of Fig. 12.9.

operating, although some control can be exercised by the use of diaphragms and by adjusting the mirrors. It is possible, with a minute pinhole, to pick out the axial mode (with amplitude distribution corresponding to Fig. 12.9). Indeed for some purposes (e.g. holography—Chapter 13) such selection is essential. When this is done, a beam of coherent light of extremely well-defined frequency results.

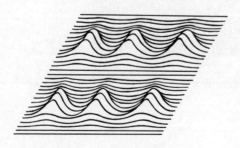

Fig. 12.11   Intensity distribution in a (2, 3) mode.

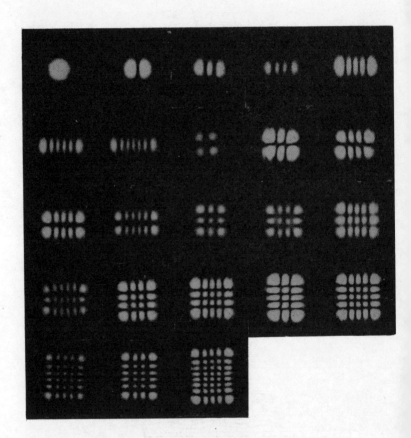

Fig. 12.12   Mode patterns obtained with a laser.

CHAPTER THIRTEEN

The laser as a tool for the physicist and technologist

The description of the laser as "a solution in search of a problem" is in the nature of a cynical comment reflecting the fact that, remarkable though its properties are, it did not immediately invade every laboratory and workshop. To some extent this is an almost inevitable reaction when a device of this kind bursts suddenly on the scientific scene. For the notable properties of the laser—its intensity, directionality and coherence—took such an enormous step forward over those for existing sources that some period of readjustment proved necessary before the implications of these advances could be fully digested. Consider, for example, the sharpness of the spectral line given by a laser compared with that of an ordinary source. The result of about a half-century's effort to produce sharper spectral lines had been that the width of such lines has been made smaller by a factor of about ten. The price paid for this improvement in sharpness was that the intensities of the sharper sources became steadily weaker. Overnight, the laser arrived with a line width a million times smaller and simultaneously at an enormous intensity. In the normal development of scientific matters, one is generally preoccupied with the kinds of problem which could be solved if one could only get a moderate improvement in one's capabilities. Although punctuated by minor advances, in understanding, techniques and methods, progress tends generally to be fairly smooth and steady. We can always think of the things which we could do with say, materials twice as strong as the present ones or with computers which are ten times as fast. However, speculation—in the complete absence of prospects—of what to do when limits change by a million times is rarely seriously indulged in. This was the situation following the arrival of the laser. It was short-lived, as one would expect, and was followed by a period of intense activity in which its remarkable properties were applied to a wide range of problems, both in the realm of "pure" science and in many areas of technology.

Perhaps we should first ask whether the arrival of the laser calls for any fundamental revision of our basic ideas in physics. The short answer is "no". The phenomenon of stimulated emission, on which the operation of the laser depends, has been allowed for in our theories of the way in which radiation and matter interact for over fifty years. The areas in which our understanding is still incomplete tend to be those associated with very high-energy physics and fundamental particle physics. The laws of physics in relation to phenomena with energies corresponding to those of the quanta of typical lasers are in general well understood and there seems at present little reason to doubt that they will stand the test of time.

Seen, however, as a tool, the laser offers enormous potentialities to the physicist for probing more deeply and with greater sensitivity into many established areas of physics, so enabling existing ideas and theories to be refined to a far higher degree than was possible hitherto.

Very many years ago, the theory was worked out which describes how radiation will react with an electron. It was shown that the chances of any interaction at all were extremely small, summed up in a cross-section of 6×10^{-25} cm^2, which indicates that if we have one electron in a square with edge 1 cm, then if we send 16×10^{23} photons through the square centimetre, only one is likely to hit the electron. When this happens, the colliding photon is deflected and, if we can detect it, we can check that scattering ("Thomson scattering") has occurred. In fact the experiment is even more difficult than may appear. It is somewhat hard to pin individual electrons down and so one has to form a beam of electrons, sending them across the light beam, and then to look for electrons scattered out of the beam. This experiment has in fact been done, although it could never have been contemplated before the enormously high intensity laser beam became available. Since then, the laser has become a much-used and powerful tool for the study of electrons in, e.g., the high energy discharges through gases (plasmas) used in attempts to produce fusion reactions in the thermonuclear energy programme. The type of discharge on which fusion hopes are pinned is highly complex. The atoms are highly ionised, so that we have a mixture of ions and electrons, moving in a complicated way and with a considerable amount of interaction going on between them. In general, an electro-magnetic wave used to explore a plasma will interact with both electrons and ions, giving a very complicated scattering be-haviour. Moreover, since such plasmas themselves give out large amounts of e.m. radiation, we have a severe problem in seeing the probing radiation against the background from the plasma—rather as though one tried to examine the sun by shining a torch at it! The extremely high intensity of the laser disposes of this problem. Although the total power of a probing laser may be very small compared with the total power radiated by the plasma, the power *at the precise laser wavelength* can be enormously higher. Thus if—say by the use of suitable colour filters—we examine only light of the laser wavelength, we are able to study the light scattered by the plasma. One further feature of this work is that it is possible to separate the effects of scattering by electrons in the plasma from that produced by the cooperative effects of electrons and ions. In the arrangement shown in Fig. 13.1, the laser light scattered in directions close to that of the ingoing beam gives information about the way in which the ions and electrons in the plasma are behaving. The light scattered sideways gives information about the electrons alone. The low-angle scattered light is found to consist partly of

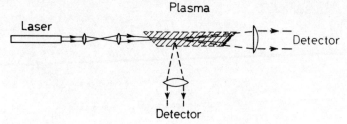

Fig. 13.1   The use of the laser for the study of plasmas.

light whose wavelength is centred on that of the laser line (but somewhat broader) and partly of light showing spectral lines either side of the main line ("satellite peaks"). The satellite peaks can give valuable information on the way in which the electrons and ions move together. The centre line tells us something about the temperature of the ions in the plasma.

In 1933 Kapitza and Dirac considered another possible way in which radiation might interact with electrons. In discussing this, they drew analogies with the way in which radiation interacts with atoms, as described in Chapter 6. The energy of the radiation may be absorbed by an atom, producing an excited atom. The latter may *either* decay spontaneously or it may be stimulated to emit by more radiation. Does this kind of thing happen to an electron? How would we know if it did? This is an intriguing problem. Suppose an electron (Fig. 13.2(a)) absorbs radiation (amount $h\nu$) from the radiation travelling from left to right and is subsequently stimulated to emit (amount $h\nu$), again by radiation travelling from left to right. The radiation emitted in the stimulated emission process travels in the same direction as that which produces the stimulated emission. Thus we had radiation energy $2\,h\nu$ in the direction AB before the scattering

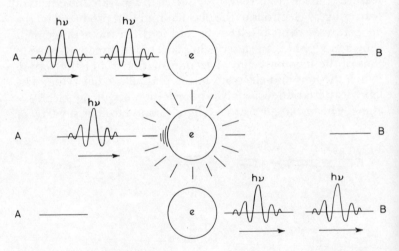

Fig. 13.2(a)   Absorption and stimulated emission of radiation by electrons. Exciting and stimulating photons in same direction.

and we have 2 *hv* in the same direction after the event. Similarly, the momenta before and after the process are $2hv/c$. Since we passionately believe in the idea that both energy and momentum are conserved, this means that the electron must end up in exactly the same state that it started. We should never know that anything had happened.

If, however, we expose our electron to a beam in which light is going in both directions (as happens if we reflect our beam from a mirror), the electron may be excited by left-to-right radiation and then be stimulated to emit by right-to-left radiation (Fig. 13.2(b)). In this case we have a net transfer of momentum to the electron. If the electron were part of a beam crossing the light beam, then it would be deflected. This is a formidably difficult experiment. When Kapitza and Dirac considered this problem, they calculated that for the most intense light and electron beams that could be produced in 1933, only one electron in every one hundred million million would be scattered. Such an experiment was quite out of the question at that time. The experiment now becomes feasible with laser intensities, with which a measurable fraction of the electron beam should be deflected. Since the amount by which the electron beam is deflected is very small (typically less than a ten-thousandth of a degree) the experiment remains extremely difficult and has not so far been done with complete certainty.

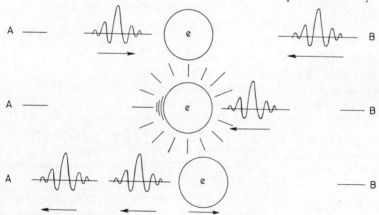

Fig. 13.2(b) Exciting and stimulating photons in opposite direction. The electron is scattered to the right.

It is, however, an essential check on whether the ideas worked out for atoms can be applied to electrons.

There are many other experiments in which radiation is scattered, e.g., by atoms and molecules, which have either become possible for the first time or have been greatly facilitated by the arrival of the laser. When a beam of light strikes a collection of atoms or molecules we expect some of it to be scattered, rather in the way that sunlight is scattered by dust in the beam. This process—known as Rayleigh scattering—is well understood and has the characteristic that the wavelength of the light scattered is exactly the same as that of the incident beam. Exactly? Strictly this applies only if the scattering atom or molecule is stationary. If the scatterer is moving, then the scattered radiation will be shifted due to the Doppler effect. Now if radiation is scattered by large, rather slow-moving molecules, the Doppler shift will not be very large—will in fact be much smaller than the normal width of the line from an ordinary source. In this case, the shift in wavelength due to the motion of the scatterer would not be measurable. In principle, such measurements *could* yield valuable information on the motion of atoms and molecules but the large width of pre-laser emission lines made Rayleigh scattering of very limited use as a tool. The very narrow linewidth of the laser, coupled with the developments of optical/electronic techniques, now enables the velocities of the scattering particles to be determined very accurately. If we scatter a beam of frequency v_0 from a particle moving with a velocity component v in the same direction, the Rayleigh-scattered frequency is $v_0(1 + v/c)$. If we mix the scattered light with some of the incident light on a photocathode, we can detect, in the photoelectric current, a frequency equal to the difference—viz. $v_0 v/c$. Thus as we know v_0 and c, we can measure v. Another way in which Rayleigh scattering may be used is to study the width of the line scattered by, e.g., a large particle in a liquid. Since the particle will be buffetted from all directions equally, it will produce a scattered line which is broader than the incident one, provided this is sufficiently sharp. Measurement of the increase in linewidth can tell us something of the motion of the particle and hence about the way in which the surrounding molecules behave. In studies of the motion of large particles in a liquid, it has been necessary in the past to infer how they move from indirect measurements. With the help of the laser, this information may now be obtained directly.

In Chapter 11, we referred to a current trend in laser development which made use of the Raman effect. This leads to the possibility of new types of laser, with wavelengths differing from those of the laser used to excite Raman spectra. Quite apart from the use of the Raman effect for producing new laser wavelengths, the laser enables an enormous extension to be made in the use of the Raman effect for its original purpose—of learning about the internal vibrations of atoms and molecules. Although the Raman effect has been used for this purpose for several decades, it has suffered from one serious limitation. Because the intensity of the wavelength-shifted lines is extremely small, it has been necessary to use very intense light sources. However, the difficulty with any conventional "monochromatic" light source is that as we make it more intense the width of the line increases. This is because, in order to produce higher intensities it is necessary to pass larger and larger currents through the lamp. The result of this is that the gas in the lamp gets hotter and so, through the Doppler effect on the emitting atoms, the range of wavelengths emitted gets larger. In many cases, much interesting information could be obtained from measurements of Raman lines which lie very close to the exciting line. With a high-current, high-pressure lamp as the exciting source, with its large associated line-width, the Raman lines are completely swamped and cannot be detected. The laser is an ideal source for this purpose. Not only is it far more intense than conventional sources, but the width of the line given out by a laser actually gets *smaller* as the power is increased. Thus the laser provides a very powerful tool for Raman spectroscopy and now forms a standard piece of hardware in the (usually chemistry) laboratory in which Raman spectroscopy is done.

In the same way that the laser has transformed the field of Raman spectroscopy, so it has enabled another, related, field to be developed. In addition to the observation of light scattered by the Raman process, we observe other lines which cannot be related to the natural frequencies of the molecules under study, as is the case with Raman lines. This second scattering process —termed Brillouin scattering—arises from the fact that a chunk of matter at ordinary temperatures consists not of stationary atoms but of atoms vibrating about an average position. Although this "thermal" vibration may appear at first sight to be a disordered behaviour, with each atom vibrating independently of its neighbours, this is by no means the case. Atoms necessarily push their neighbours around as they vibrate and we need to think of the whole mass of material when describing its thermal behaviour. We can do this by imagining the material to display the effect of waves—acoustic (sound) waves—running back and forth through the material in all directions. Unlike the electromagnetic waves which characterise light, these waves involve the actual displacement of whole atoms from their average positions in the substance considered. What will be the amplitudes and frequencies of the waves present? This will depend in a very complicated way on the structure of the material. In fact, information on these aspects of the acoustic waves in a solid can provide invaluable guidance on its behaviour and properties.

Suppose, now, the beam from a laser impinges on a solid (or liquid). The electric field in the light wave will influence the electrons of the atoms in the material. If all the atoms were stationary, then Rayleigh and Raman scattering would occur, with the results as discussed earlier. When, however, the atoms are moving in a way corresponding to waves moving through them, the amplitude of any scattered light will be affected (modulated) by the acoustic waves in the specimen. In the same way that modulation of a radio wave produces sidebands, of different frequency from that of the carrier, so the effects of acoustic waves in a solid or liquid can produce sidebands, or Brillouin-scattered radiation, from an incident laser beam. By studying the Brillouin-shifted light, we are able to deduce how the corresponding acoustic waves in the material behave. This can be immensely important because, although we can study the behaviour of some acoustic waves directly, we can do this only for certain limited ranges of frequency. Our understanding of the acoustic spectrum is a good deal more limited than of the electromagnetic spectrum—rather as though we were investigating the latter using our eyes only. We should be blissfully unaware of, e.g., the radio-frequency region in this case.

Many of the techniques used to exploit the laser, in the examples given above, make use of the fact that the light from a laser is coherent, as discussed in Chapter 5. There is another field, known as "holography", or "wavefront reconstruction", which has developed extremely rapidly since the arrival of the laser. The technique was first proposed twelve years before the arrival of the laser, but little progress could be made because of the absence of powerful coherent light sources.

Holography is a method of producing optical images in three dimensions and with full perspective, as distinct from conventional photography which inevitably produces only a two-dimensional representation of an object. (Although stereoscopic photography produces a three-dimensional effect, this is restricted to a reconstruction of a scene viewed from a pair of fixed cameras.)

Let us first consider how a photograph would reconstruct an image of several small points of light at approximately (but not exactly) the same distance from a lens, as shown in Fig. 13.3. If

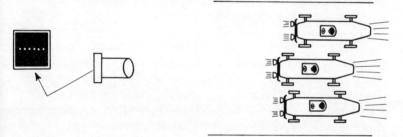

Fig. 13.3 Formation of image of several points at very slightly different distances from a lens.

the sources have all the same intensity, the photograph will consist of a number of similar spots of light, with no indication that they are not all in the same plane. Remembering, however, that light is a wave-motion, we may note that crests and troughs from the light from different sources will not necessarily arrive in step. Whether or not a crest arrives at a given instant will depend on the distance from light source to plate. If we have two sources emitting waves which are in step (i.e. are coherent) but whose distances from the photographic plate differ by one half wavelength (Fig. 13.4), the crest of the wave from one

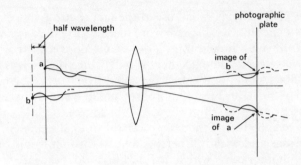

Fig. 13.4   The photographs of two points of light whose distances from the plate differ by a half-wavelength would be similar.

source will meet the plate at the same time as the trough from the other. The plate however is aware only that light waves are arriving at each point and it blackens accordingly. It is not able to distinguish the two waves—i.e. it cannot record the *phase* of the wave. Now it is the phase of the wave which provides some information on the position of the source of light. Information on the size and shape of an illuminated object is contained in the amplitude *and* phase of light scattered from it. We cannot hope to reconstruct a true copy of the object unless we record both amplitude and phase of the waves from all points of the object. How can this be done when the photographic plate cannot distinguish phase? The answer is that if a coherent light source is available phase information *can* be recorded if the light scattered from the object is mixed with a part of the wave used to illuminate the object (a "reference wave"). For consider the effect of adding a reference wave to the light from the two sources shown in Fig. 13.4. If we add a wave whose crest coincides with that from the upper source, the result will be a large intensity and hence a strong blackening of the plate. For the lower source, the crest of the reference wave coincides with the trough of the wave from the source: the waves tend to cancel so that very little blackening occurs. By this means, therefore, the two waves may be distinguished and phase information obtained. This then is the principle underlying holography—the recording of phase information by the interference of light scattered by an object with that of a *coherent* reference wave.

The combined amplitude and phase information are recorded

on a photographic plate, resulting in a hologram. This is made in one of a number of ways, one of which is illustrated in Fig. 13.5. The light from a laser is made parallel by a lens system and part of it illuminates the object. The remainder is reflected by a mirror and the two sets of waves strike the photographic plate. Here, a complicated interference pattern forms, depending on the form of the object. (If the object is a flat reflecting surface, the interference pattern consists of a set of parallel fringes: if a small dot, then a set of rings forms on the plate.)

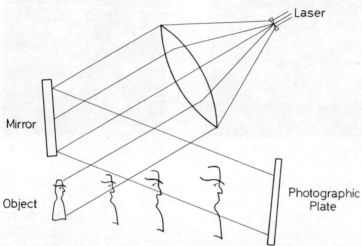

Fig. 13.5   One of the ways of producing a hologram. (The wave scattered by the object is more complicated than as shown.)

If the photographic plate is developed and illuminated with a wave similar to that used as a reference wave in making the hologram, then an observer sees a complete, three-dimensional reconstruction of the original object. As he moves his head, the reconstruction changes so as to present the different views which would be seen if he were looking at the object itself. An illustration, made from photographs of a reconstruction by a hologram, is shown in Fig. 13.6. The three pictures correspond to different viewing directions through the hologram. The effect of perspective is clearly seen.

The crucial feature of a light source for holography is that the light must be coherent over a reasonable length. This is because one relies on interference between waves which have travelled different distances, as must inevitably be the case if a three-dimensional object is to be recorded. Conventional light-sources of adequate power produce waves which cannot interfere, in the way required for holography, if the different waves (source-object-plate and source-reference mirror plate) travel by paths which differ by more than a small fraction of a millimetre.

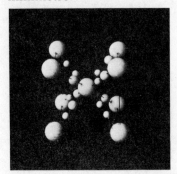 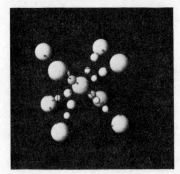

Fig. 13.6   Reconstructions made from a single hologram, viewed from different directions.

An intriguing feature of the hologram is that the information relating to the whole of the illuminated object is spread over the whole hologram plate. Thus if a plate is broken in half, the reconstructed image may be seen through either half. The fact that an image, in the normal sense, does *not* form on the plate itself means that the perfection of the reconstruction is not seriously impaired by scratches and dust on the plate. In contrast, scratches on a conventional photographic negative inevitably result in scratches on the resulting print.

Several properties of holograms make them of great importance for many technological and engineering applications. One such feature is that very many holograms can be stored on a single plate. Provided the direction of the reference beam relative to the plate is changed between exposures, the superposed hologram patterns are not confused. Reconstructions are formed only when the developed plate is illuminated by a beam *in the appropriate direction*. Thus if a hologram containing many patterns is rotated in the path of a fixed beam, the observer sees the many reconstructions appearing sequentially. In this way, considerable amounts of information—e.g. in a data storage system—can be stored in a single plate and can be retrieved simply by illuminating at an appropriate angle.

One potentially powerful technique which has emerged in the development of holography is that which enables small deformations of an object to be studied, or small differences to be revealed between the dimensions of a master object and a copy. Suppose a hologram is made of an object which has been accurately made to certain specified dimensions and suppose that it is desired to compare with this the size and shape of, say, mass-produced copies. This can be done by making a hologram of the "perfect" master copy, illuminating the hologram so as to produce a reconstruction, which again will be perfect, and then placing a test object exactly in register with the holographically reconstructed image. If the test object is *exactly* the same size and if it occupies precisely the space where the reconstruction lies, then only a single object (or reconstruction—or both!) is seen. If, however, the object differs slightly in size from the master (and hence from the reconstruction) then interference fringes are seen crossing the object (Fig. 13.7). Each successive fringe from a given point of reference indicates a difference in size of one half-wavelength between the test object and the master. Since the helium-neon laser is often used for this purpose, this results in a technique able to compare sizes of objects to within about 0·0003 mm. Of particular importance is that no preparation of the test object is required. Alternatively, since two or more patterns may be stored on the same plate, holograms of the master and test object may be recorded on a single plate. The reconstruction will then itself show fringes indicating any difference of size.

The direction in which the reconstructed image from a hologram is seen depends on the wavelength of the light used for the recording or reconstruction process. (These need not be the same.) The colour by which the reconstruction is seen is clearly that of the light used for the reconstruction. By suitable choice of illuminating lasers, of different colours, and of reconstructing wavelengths, we may in fact store—on a black-and-white photographic plate—holographic patterns which when illuminated simultaneously with, say, red, green and blue lasers, yield a holographic reconstruction in full colour.

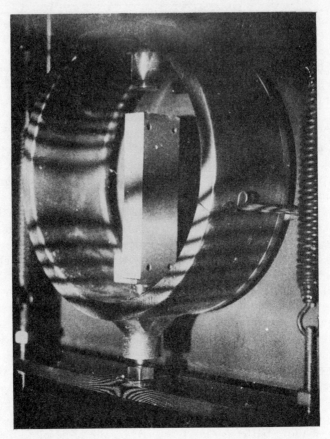

Fig. 13.7 Fringes showing difference in size between an object and a holographic reconstruction.

The likely applications of holography in technology are too numerous to discuss in detail. In addition to the comparison of "static" samples, holography with high-power pulsed lasers may be used to study the shape or deformation of bodies travelling at high speed. Thus a ruby laser pulse lasting only a hundred millionth of a second is easily produced: in this time, an object moving at ten times the speed of sound moves only three hundredths of a millimetre. Thus the reconstruction (which can be done with a continuous laser) would show no blurring, but would provide a "frozen" picture of the object, even at this speed.

The use of the laser in holography is one of the examples of the way in which information carried by waves of light can be handled. When we look at an object (or an image produced by a lens system), we are taking part in a data-processing operation. Light scattered from the object carries information about it and this data is observed by the eye and processed by the brain. We can see in a very simple way how the information being carried in this system could be processed in such a way as to pick out particular characteristics of the data being presented. Thus if we simply put in a filter of a given colour, the parts of the object with that colour will be clearly seen while the remainder will appear indistinct (or will not be seen at all if the colours are sufficiently differentiated). From this very crude concept, data processing systems of great complexity have emerged and in many cases their development has been made possible by the development of the laser. Could we, for example, design a system so that, when a complicated object is observed, the presence of one particular kind of detail only is detected? One thinks of two immediate uses for such a system. In the regular screening of patients for certain kinds of disease it is necessary to search for particular kinds of cell in specimens of, e.g., saliva or other secretions. In the case of diseases which are extremely rare but which are nevertheless so serious as to warrant considerable effort at detection, this problem involves the formidable task of observing enormous numbers of microscope slides, each with a large number of cells on them, and for which perhaps only one in a thousand has any abnormality. This can be done by training observers, who then pass endless days peering down microscopes in a way which can perhaps at best be of limited fascination. A second application arises in the military field where it is required, from reconaissance photographs of the enemy's territory, to identify particular military installations such as missile sites. Since such photographs will generally be from high-flying aircraft or satellites, the image of such installations will occupy only a minute part of the whole photograph. This, as with the medical problem referred to above, is a problem in pattern recognition. One needs a way of telling, quickly, whether, from a large amount of information presented, any is present with certain known characteristic features. This may be located anywhere over a photographic plate (or microscope field of view) and may be in any orientation.

To see how this can be tackled, we digress for a moment to examine the way in which a lens system forms an image. The formation of the image of a real object with white light is somewhat complicated (variety of detail and range of colours) so let us take a very simple, regular object—a piece of transparent material with grooves across it—and a monochromatic source of light. Suppose the grooves are such (Fig. 13.8) that the surface of the plate forms a regular sine wave pattern and imagine this plate illuminated by a parallel beam of monochromatic light. In this case, we observe three beams emerging from the plate, one being the continuation of the illuminating beam and the other two equally inclined on either side of the central beam. (There are in fact beams in other directions, but these are extremely weak compared with those described above.) If we put a lens beyond the plate then we can produce an image of the plate on a screen—provided, that is, we do not put the lens so far from the plate that the two sideways diffracted beams miss the lens altogether. If however we explore the region between lens and image, using a ground glass screen, we find a place where the three beams emerging from the plate all come to a focus, giving three spots, as shown at A, B, C in Fig. 13.8. There is practically no light anywhere else in this (focal) plane and if we put in a screen with three holes, coinciding with the diffraction spots, we should see no difference in the image. We can consider the image itself as being formed by the effect of inter-

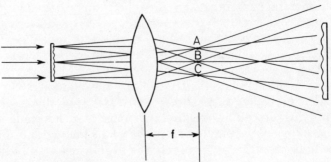

Fig. 13.8   Formation of image of a sinusoidal grating object.

ference between the light beams emerging from the points A, B and C in the focal plane of the lens.

If the grating object of Fig. 13.8 is rotated about the lens axis, then the spots A and C rotate: they occur in a direction perpendicular to that of the rulings on the object grating. An important property from the pattern recognition angle, however, is that if the grating object is moved about in its own plane (but without rotation) the positions of the spots A and C *do not* change. The intensity of the spots A and C will depend on the area of the grating present, but not on its position. Thus if with a complicated object we observe any light at A and C, this indicates that the object somewhere contains detail with the form of the grating shown in Fig. 13.8.

The light which is focused at points such as A in Fig. 13.8 is that which has left the object in a certain direction. The direction of the light diffracted by a grating depends on the spacing of the rulings on the grating and on the wavelength. For a given wavelength, the finer the grating, the larger will be the angle of diffraction. It is convenient to think of the number of lines per centimetre of the grating as a "spatial frequency", in the same way that a time frequency is the number of cycles in one second. We see then that each point in the focal plane of a lens producing an image corresponds to a particular spatial frequency which occurs in the detail of the object. Although the distribution of light in the focal plane bears not the slightest resemblance to that in the object, there is a complete correspondence between them. (The distribution of light in the focal plane of the lens is termed the Fourier Transform of the distribution in the object.)

Suppose now we take a complicated object, form an image, as in Fig. 13.9, and place a mask with holes at A, B and C in the

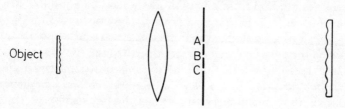

Fig. 13.9   If a screen allows only light through A, B, C to pass, a sinusoidal image, similar to that of Fig. 13.8, forms.

focal plane of the lens. If the object contains any detail resembling the grating shown in Fig. 13.8, this will produce light at A and C which will, together with that from B, form an image of that detail.

This lengthy discussion may have an air of unreality about it. We are generally concerned with an object which is vastly more complicated than the simple sine grating considered above. In fact the arguments can still be applied, for if we superpose a suitable selection of gratings, of different amplitudes and spacing and in different orientations, we can in fact produce a distribution of light corresponding to that of any object. Since under all conditions of interest two light waves whose amplitudes separately at a given point are a_1 and a_2 produce, when acting together, an amplitude $a_1 + a_2$, any argument we use about a single grating can be extended to the case of a whole collection of gratings. Let us go back, then, to our original problem—of pattern recognition. We want to identify a feature of known shape in a photograph or object with a lot of (to us irrelevant) information on it. We can determine what light distribution the feature of interest would produce in the focal plane of the lens. We make a filter, to place in the focal plane, which lets just this kind of light distribution through. If, now, with our complex object, we put in such a filter, light will come through *if* detail corresponding to the sought-after feature is present. Since the intensity distribution in the Fourier transform of the feature does not depend on its position in the object, this type of recognition system will detect a wanted feature anywhere in the field of the object.

The part played by the laser in this kind of application is important. Although in principle this kind of thing can be done without a laser, the enormously greater intensity of the laser turns the method from one of limited, academic importance to one of considerable practical power. The Fourier Transform of an object in an optical system serves as a useful "fingerprint". Indeed the very problem of searching through the vast numbers of fingerprints on file in criminal investigation departments may well be alleviated by just such a method as this. The general point is that in many circumstances features must be distinguished against a large background of irrelevant or redundant information. The use of the Fourier Transform offers such a possibility. Its implementation in a system using lasers and the associated hardware of detectors and automatic devices is already under way in many areas. The above are simple examples of the way in which automated data-handling and processing can be achieved with lasers: this field is developing at an extremely rapid rate.

Closely associated with any developments concerned with data handling are those in the fields of electronics. The revolution which has occurred over the last twenty years in the electronics field is on the same scale as that produced by the laser in the field of optics. The successful development of the transistor marked the first major step which transformed the electronic scene and marked the demise of the thermionic valve for all but a specialised range of purposes. The transistor— lighter, smaller and requiring simpler power supplies—has enabled electronic technology to move into new fields even if some of the social aspects of the transistor radio appear as dubious signs of progress. The next major step in electronic development takes us into the realm of microcircuits, in which minute slices of semiconductor are delicately fashioned in a way that produces complicated circuitry of the kind hitherto requiring whole arrays of aluminium chassis, valves, resistors, capacitors and yards of wire.

The coherence of the laser enables very precise measurements to be made over much longer distances than hitherto. The facility thus emerges of precise calibration of such things as machine tools. An example of the precision attainable is shown in Fig. 13.10 giving the error in the calibration of the scale of a jig-boring machine. Errors as small as a two-thousandth of a millimetre are readily detected. Furthermore the laser may be employed to control machine tools, thus making them independent of the accuracy of the scale of the machine. Movements of the cutting edges of the tool are controlled directly in terms of the wavelength of the laser, which is constant to an extremely high degree.

On a much larger scale, the lasers may be used in surveying instruments. One development of interest here is the use of the laser to study the relative movement of different parts of the earth's surface. It seems likely that such measurements may be applied to the study of earthquake areas and may enable ad-

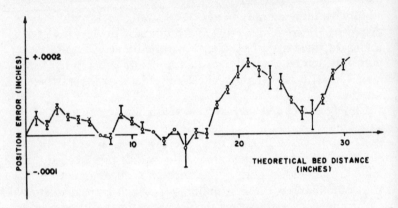

Fig. 13.10   Calibration curve for a jig-boring machine.

vanced warning of earthquakes to be obtained. One intriguing possibility here concerns the question of continental drift. For many years, the theory that the continents of Africa and South America are drifting apart (and were indeed at one time joined together) has been hotly debated. The original suggestion was made in the 1920s but was subsequently rejected. Since the 1950s, however, further evidence has accumulated lending support to the idea. Thus from studies of the state of the Earth's magnetic field over a long period, it is impossible to define a location for the magnetic pole unless continental drift has occurred. From consideration of the Earth's thermal conductivity, it is difficult to see how the heat generated within the Earth (from radioactivity) could be dissipated without a convection such as a drift would imply. Furthermore, a study of the geological age of the rocks on the north-west region of South America and of those along the Ghana/Dahomey/Nigeria region of Africa reveals two adjacent regions, one of rocks about 2,000 million years old and one of only 500 million years. When the two continents are fitted together, the line of demarcation between the two regions appears continuous. One is moved, therefore, to speculate on whether it would be possible to detect directly the widening gap. The rate of drift is expected to be of the order of a few centimetres per year. There appear two possible ways of doing this, with the help of a pulsed laser. Simultaneous measurement of the distance from points on the two continents to an orbiting satellite yields results for which the standard deviation for a single measurement is of the order 1 m. For a reasonable number of repeated readings, therefore, mean distances accurate to better than ± 10 cm should be attainable. A second method is to make use of the Earth's natural satellite, the Moon, whose orbit is now known to a high degree of accuracy. In this case, too, an accuracy of ± 10 cm should be attainable. It seems possible, therefore, that by making such measurements over a period of about ten years, direct evidence of drift could be obtained.

In the field of communication, the laser offers an enormous potential. Because of its coherence, radiation from a laser resembles that from a radio transmitter rather than that from a conventional, incoherent, light source. If the same techniques are evolved for impressing signals on laser beams as are used for radio waves, lasers can clearly be used for communication. The amount of information which can be carried on an electro-magnetic wave increases as the frequency increases. Roughly, one can say that the number of channels of bandwidth f that can be imposed on a carrier wave of frequency F is simply F/f. To carry sound radio, a bandwidth f of about 5,000 cycles per second is needed. Since the frequency of a typical laser beam is 10^{15} cycles per second, we see that we could in principle carry more than ten thousand million such programmes on a single laser beam. The technology necessary to realise this enormous capacity has not yet evolved. Nevertheless even at the present time the capability exists of carrying enormously more information on a laser beam than can be transmitted along radio beams. Moreover the greater directionality of the laser means that less power is needed to communicate between two stations.

A serious drawback to the laser for terrestrial communication is that laser beams are stopped by fog or cloud. They are likely however to have a significant role to play in space communication. Even for terrestrial communication, however, the potential of the laser is so enormous that active consideration is being given to the use either of pipes or of glass fibres as a means of overcoming the atmospheric difficulty. At present, the prospects of making glass fibres sufficiently perfect to enable them to be used over long distances seem formidable. We may recall, however, that at the early stages of the development of semi-conductors, the technological difficulties of making materials of the very high purity required seemed daunting. Within a few years, however, these had been solved and the transistor has become a cheap and common piece of electronic hardware.

It is certain that the field of computers will make great strides as a result of the invention of the laser. In particular, we can expect rapid developments in the use of optical/electronic (or "opto-electronic") methods of data handling. One such example is in the use of materials which can be coloured by exposure to a laser beam. Such materials are termed "photochromic". If a crystal of this type is exposed to a scanning laser beam, similar to the scanning electron beam on a television tube, then by varying the intensity of the laser beam a series of coloured dots may be written on the crystal. Thus information, in the form of the "scale-of-two" used in computer memories, may be stored in such a crystal. By the use of a weaker beam, the information may be read out of such a memory. The interest in this form of storage derives from the fact that the laser beam can be focused to a very small diameter, so that an enormous number of dots may be written in this way on a small area of crystal. A further important feature is that materials exist for which dots may be "written" with a laser beam of one wavelength and may be erased by light from a laser of different wavelength. This is of great importance for an information store which needs to be updated. The "erase" beam is used to remove out-of-date information, which can then be replaced by new information on the "write" beam. One of many applications of a facility of this type is that of airline bookings, where the stored information has continually to be changed.

Looking still further ahead, one can see that each of the dots on such a crystal may in fact be a hologram, perhaps of a whole page of a book. The ultimate shape of the library of the future may be radically different from the present one. The printed page gives place to arrays of photochromic crystals which are scanned, on command from a telegraphed signal from the reader (in a neighbouring city). The appropriate page hologram is selected and reconstructed on a television tube which is scanned and transmitted—via a laser fibre, or a pipe system, to the reader. The incoming signal is then used to produce a printed sheet on the reader's receiving equipment unless, that is, the reader merely wishes to consult the page at the time of viewing, in which case he would simply read the page from a television screen.

It must be admitted that this highly fanciful concept would require some radical changes in our habits. The crucial point is that the technology to enable this to be done is very near. There appears to be a case for a critical appraisal of our present methods of information-handling.

In this chapter a small selection of examples has been given of the vast number of actual and potential applications to science and technology. There are a host of others—machining and cutting of (any) materials; spectroscopy of minute samples produced by laser pulses; automatic micromachining of electronic circuits; meteorological studies by laser scattering; control of chemical reactions by lasers; laser gyroscopes; flow measurement by measurement of Doppler shift; seismometry; automatic pattern recognition—the list is endless. Perhaps one should mention finally an application which could have particularly far-reaching consequences. It is one which arises from the fact that, by focusing a high-energy laser beam, one can produce plasmas of very high temperature. For the operation of a fusion reaction (hydrogen bomb) a very high temperature is required. At the moment, the conditions necessary for fusion can be achieved only by the explosion of a fission bomb. A fission bomb is an extremely complex device, requiring not only highly advanced technology but industrial resources on a very large scale. By contrast, high-power lasers require only modest resources. If the stage is reached whereby fusion devices can be operated by lasers then the balance of military power could shift abruptly from a small number of nations with vast resources to a much wider range of governments and even to private organisations. This situation may not be as far away as seems to be thought at this time.

CHAPTER FOURTEEN

The laser in biology and medicine

The notice which is prominently displayed on the doors of laboratories containing lasers, namely

DANGER
LASER IN USE
BEAM CAN CAUSE
PERMANENT EYE DAMAGE

provides a strong indication of one of the effects of laser radiation on human tissue. The powers available in present lasers are such that the most stringent safety precautions are required in their use. The hazard of the high-power carbon dioxide laser —which will burn a hole through a firebrick in seconds—is an obvious one so far as danger to humans is concerned. Less obvious is the potential harm that can result from looking at say, a helium-neon laser beam of only one thousandth of a watt. Because the lens of the eye focuses the beam on to a minute spot on the retina, the intensity of illumination on the retinal cells could easily be high enough to cause damage. As we shall see later in this chapter, this aspect of lasers and eyes can in fact be put to good use in dealing with a certain type of eye disorder.

What are the ways in which laser radiation will affect biological material? There appear to be four important mechanisms which can operate. First, the high intensity in a laser beam may produce heating, so producing a burn or even complete volatilisation of the material. Secondly, the laser beam may generate high-intensity acoustic (sound or ultrasonic) waves which may not only damage material in the neighbourhood of the laser shot, but may propagate to more distant regions. Thirdly, the large electric field associated with the intense beam may affect the biological material. Fourthly, a pressure wave may spread out from the point of impact. Our present understanding of many of these effects is at a very primitive level and much basic work is needed before many potentially useful applications of lasers in the medical field can be fully exploited.

Before discussing the application of lasers to a whole living system, let us first look at the way in which they may be used at a most basic level—in the study of cells.

Two features of the laser make it a possible tool for the study of living cells. One is the power available and the other is that the laser beam can be focussed—by using a microscope in reverse—to an extremely fine spot. The size attainable is much smaller than that of a typical cell and offers an intriguing possibility of learning about the functional relationships of different parts of a cell. Basically, a cell consists of a nucleus surrounded by a volume of cytoplasm. The cytoplasm contains a vast variety of minute features—of the order of a thousandth of a millimetre across—whose detailed role in the processes going on is not well understood. Since a laser beam may be focussed to spots of this size, it is possible to damage selectively the individual cell components and to study the effect of such damage on the subsequent cell behaviour. With conventional sources of light it has never been possible to produce a sufficiently localised spot to enable such selective studies to be made. Since the cytoplasm is transparent to visible laser radiation, it is unaffected in the process. Moreover no damage is done to the cell wall, as occurs if attempts are made to interfere with the inner parts of the cell by using probes.

In the field of embryology, the use of a laser in this general way could lead to a better understanding of the mechanism of transmission of hereditary diseases. In the development of a complete organism from a fertilised ovum, a "watershed" is reached at the point where the descended cells take on specialised functions. Up to that point an apparently complete organism can develop even if some cells are damaged or destroyed.

Beyond that stage, damage to cells results in a defective organism. The feasibility of producing controllable damage to individual cells represents a significant development in the methods available for work of this kind.

On a coarser scale, the laser can be used simply as a brute-force tool to produce controllable damage to parts of an organism. An application in which the laser proves useful in this way is the testing of anticoagulants, designed to suppress blood-clotting. Such testing requires a method of creating clots in a *reproducible* manner and the laser provides just such a facility.

In certain cases, the selective destruction of unwanted tissue is required—e.g. in the removal of dark, pigmented areas of tissue (melanomata). In this case, the high absorption of the abnormal tissue for laser radiation means that pigmented cells can be destroyed by a laser flash at an intensity which produces no damage to normal tissue. Melanomata have been successfully dealt with in this manner. There are some aspects of this work which are not yet well understood, especially those concerning the behaviour of growths which are only partially destroyed by a laser flash. In some cases, regression of the remaining, untreated, part occurs whereas in others no such effect is observed. Nevertheless, there are promising indications that laser treatment of melanomata and of small tumours may be extremely effective. Although there has been insufficient time for long-term effects to be observed, there have been no unwanted after-effects over periods of two or three years.

To go one stage further, we may consider the possible role of the laser in surgery, as an alternative to the scalpel for producing incisions. The intensities available in present lasers are more than adequate to produce incisions, by the simple process of burning. Such burning is, however, with a focussed laser beam, extremely localised. Moreover, the heating effect of the beam used in this way seals the severed blood-vessels so that little or no bleeding results. By careful control of the laser power, the depth of such incisions is easily regulated. Since no contact is involved with an instrument, problems of sterilisation do not arise and indeed the high temperature produced at the incised organ or tissue itself ensures sterile conditions.

One question to be answered in connection with the use of the laser in this way relates to the subsequent healing of the incision.

At the time of writing, the results appear highly encouraging. Sub-cutaneous tissue appears to heal in exactly the same way that occurs with conventional surgery. The situation over surface tissue is less clear but it is possible that the optimum conditions—of beam intensity and cutting rate—have not yet been established. Where large blood vessels are present, some loss of blood is observed but this is very much smaller than that resulting from conventional surgery. There is also evidence that the clotting time for laser incisions is far less than that for scalpel treatment.

The laser is easily able to drill holes in bone and has been used successfully, on animals, to remove sections of bone from the skull, as is needed for brain operations. It can excise brain tissue bloodlessly, with no apparent effect on the adjacent tissue and so may well have a part to play in the treatment of brain tumours. Since the majority of brain tumours are malignant, the need to minimise bleeding (with consequent risk of spreading malignant cells to other parts) is paramount. Another tumour problem which may be susceptible to laser surgery is that of removing tumours from the spinal cord. Although these are generally non-malignant, their removal by conventional means is generally a bloody business. The obscuration produced by heavy bleeding increases the risk of damage to the spinal cord during the operation.

In experiments of this kind discussed above, continuous wave lasers using argon, carbon dioxide and neodymium in YAG have been used. Different behaviour is observed from one to another, reflecting the difference in the tissue characteristics at the different wavelengths involved. Too little basic data is as yet available to enable a pre-judgment to be made as to which laser will be most useful for any particular task.

In the bloodless removal of cancerous growths (or indeed in any treatment involving the use of laser radiation) the vital question arises as to whether the effect of the radiation itself could result in abnormal cell development. If it is assumed that the kind of abnormalities which arise in irradiation by very high energy particles necessarily involve the direct action of a high-energy quantum, then there seems little likelihood that similar effects would arise from laser irradiation. Although the total energy delivered to a piece of tissue may be large, the energy of the individual radiation quanta is low. If, for example, cell damage of the kind under discussion required quanta of energy, say 20,000 eV, then this would need 10,000 laser quanta to arrive virtually simultaneously at the cell and the chances of such a multi-photon process occurring are vanishingly small. However, it would be idle to pretend that we understand the reasons for the development of abnormal cells sufficiently well to be perfectly confident. Extreme caution is therefore being exercised in this work. To date there is no evidence that abnormal cell growth occurs in laser-irradiated tissue.

One of the earliest medical applications of the laser was that of dealing with the detached retina. In this condition, which may result from a heavy blow or from certain diseases, the layer of retinal cells becomes separated from the choroid. If not treated, the condition leads to complete blindness. Reattachment may be effected by laying the patient on his back, so that the retina sinks down in the correct position, and by firing a low-energy pulsed laser into the eye in the appropriate direction. The retina is effectively "spot-welded" back in place. Since the laser spot (focussed by the lens in the eye) is very small, only few retinal cells are damaged in the process. An example of such a weld is shown in Fig. 14.1, which shows a section through a rabbit's eye treated in this way. Further interesting features of this method are (1) that since the laser flash used lasts less than a thousandth of a second, extremely immobilisation of the patient is unnecessary, (2) the duration of the process is less than the minimum required for a stimulus to produce a pain sensation and (3) since no surgery is involved, no problems of sterility or infection arise.

The idea of repairing detached retinas by the use of an intense light flash is not new. Before the arrival of the laser, this operation was carried out using a high-intensity xenon arc source. Because of the lack of directionality of this type of source and of its incoherence, it is not possible to produce an intense, highly localised spot on the retina. Typically, a flash delivering about 3 joules of energy and of duration about 1 sec is used with the xenon source. Although a high success rate is achieved, the xenon arc method inevitably produces damage to rather many retinal cells and in a few per cent of cases treated, this damage is such as to produce severe impairment of vision. In part, this

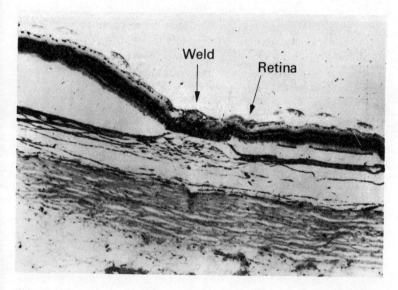

Fig. 14.1   Section of retina of rabbit's eye, welded by laser coagulator.

stems from the long duration of the pulse required to produce coagulation. During this time, a significant amount of heat diffuses away from the weld region, with resultant damage to cells around, as well as at the focus of the weld site. With a ruby laser source it is found to be possible to produce satisfactory welds with energies as small as a few thousandths of a joule, in pulses lasting only a thousandth of a second. Such welds are only a small fraction of a millimetre in diameter and produce no noticeable effect on vision. Moreover, the strength of several small welds over a given area of retina is very much greater than that of a single, large weld, such as is produced by the xenon arc. This is because the strength of the weld depends on the total length of the peripheries of the welded regions. In the case of laser welds observed over a period of a year or two, the layer supporting the retina (the pigment epithelium) is found to have grown over the whole area of the weld. In contrast, the xenon arc treatment destroys the pigment epithelium over too large an area for re-growth to be possible.

The early evidence for the effectiveness of laser retinal treatment is highly encouraging. Not only have such welds proved to be permanent, but the ability of the eye to distinguish fine detail (the visual acuity) is found to return to its normal value.

It is too early to comment on very long-term effects of laser retinal surgery. The apparent absence of any harmful effects is such as to suggest that this may prove a very significant advance in the treatment of this type of disorder.

It is clear that the application of lasers to the studies of molecular structures can be extended to the realm of biological materials. The use of the laser for Raman spectroscopy has already been mentioned. For biological molecules, Raman spectroscopy has powerful and important possibilities. One of the standard methods of studying molecules is that of determining how the absorption of infra-red radiation varies with the wavelength. This method has two limitations, both of which may be very serious for biological materials. On the one hand, the infra-red absorption spectrum of a biological molecule may be extremely complex—so much so that it may be impossible to interpret. On the other, the absorption of water for some infra-red wavelengths is very heavy indeed—so heavy that it becomes impossible to study materials in aqueous solution. Raman spectra do not share these serious drawbacks and this technique may well be applicable where infra-red methods fail.

The need for caution and for extensive testing of a new device in the medical field, in order to be certain that no harmful side-effects ensue, means that this introduction of lasers in this field will be gradual. It already is clear, however, that the laser has much to contribute—both directly, as in the examples discussed above, and indirectly through the developments in other technologies.

CHAPTER FIFTEEN

The impact of lasers in the future

It may seem presumptuous to single out one of the many technological developments in the middle of the twentieth century and to speculate on the kind of impact which it is likely to make in the future. At the same time it is apparent from the topics discussed in the last few chapters that the advances which the laser makes possible are likely to be so dramatic that there appear good reasons for believing that its influence will be felt over an area vastly wider than that of the scientific and technological fields in which it is being developed.

In this concluding chapter we shall examine a number of fields of human endeavour to see whether any significant changes are likely to occur in the foreseeable future as a result of the emergence of this remarkable device. Inevitably some of the speculations will have a crystal ball quality about them. Inevitably, too, some of the tentative forecasts will prove wrong in time. We shall see, however, that in certain areas issues are raised which will require (or indeed already require) fundamental re-thinking.

Space travel

Let us look first at the field which currently looms large in man's interest, that of space exploration. The success achieved in ferrying men to our nearest neighbour in the Solar System must surely raise the question of more distant exploration. We first examine the extent to which such developments are possible and then ask what part, if any, the laser can be expected to play in this field.

The briefest examination of the prospects of exploration into space suffices to show that we shall never (at least on a round-trip basis within the human life-span) be able to venture far into the space which we so readily observe. It is no accident that our familiar unit of length, the metre, or kilometre, proves an inconvenient one in which to measure distances in space. While we are discussing lunar expeditions, the kilometre is not too impractical a measure since the earth-moon distance is around 380,000 km. Even the earth-sun distance, of 150,000,000 km lies within the grasp of our imagination (although even this is arguable). Anything beyond this requires a more convenient unit. There are two such units in use, the light-year and the parsec. The light-year is the distance which light travels in vacuum in one year and is nearly six million million miles.*

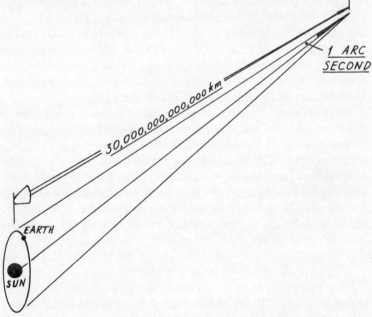

Fig. 15.1

* An English billion is 10^{12}: an American billion 10^{9}. To minimise confusion the term billion will be avoided.

Astronomers generally prefer to work with the parsec, which is the distance at which a line equal in length to the radius of the earth's solar orbit subtends an angle of one second of arc (Fig. 15.1). The parsec is 3×10^{13} km—or thirty million million km.

A few brief comments will serve to indicate the immensity of the system of stars and galaxies which we can observe. Our own solar system extends over a diameter of a few thousand million kilometres and forms one of perhaps ten thousand million such systems in our own galaxy, which is roughly disc-shaped and about twenty-five thousand parsecs in diameter. Our nearest neighbour in this system is about 1·3 parsecs away—the star Alpha Centauri. Our galaxy is one of about 10–100 thousand million such galaxies, occupying the region of space which we can observe, which extends to a few hundred million parsecs. Although we cannot pretend that this is a very definite figure, depending as it does on a number of assumptions, it should not be too far out. Thus the light (or radiation generally) which we receive from distant parts of the observable universe started on its journey to us several hundred million years ago. On our present beliefs, the velocity of light represents a limiting speed beyond which we cannot accelerate material bodies so that we can see no way of physically travelling in times less than that taken for light to make the journey.

Although our own galaxy is one of an enormous number distributed through space, even its size is such that we have no foreseeable prospects of visiting any of it. The round-trip time for a light signal between our own solar system and the most distant part of our galaxy is about seventy thousand years. What of the closer regions? Is there any prospect of paying a visit to Alpha Centauri, at 4×10^{13} km (1·3 parsecs, or 4·3 light years) distance away? A cursory examination of the powers available with present-day forms of rocket suffices to show that such a journey is completely beyond the scope of such devices. Let us imagine, however, that nuclear-powered rockets become a reality and consider what would be involved in making a round-trip to Alpha Centauri in, say, about 10 years. If the journey is made at a speed of two-thirds of the velocity of light, then the elapsed time for the astronaut would be about 10 years (although his earth-bound relatives would record an interval of

13 years for his absence—a consequence of relativity). In fact, we should need time to accelerate the rocket to this speed, a time determined by the fact that the human frame does not take kindly to excessive acceleration. At the (uncomfortable) level of 6g (six times the acceleration due to gravity at the earth's surface), this velocity would be reached within about a year. Although the human body can withstand such an acceleration for a short time, we have no means of knowing whether such a long continuous exposure could be tolerated. Supposing this to be possible, what kind of energy would be required for such a venture? If we assume that for a ten-year journey the rocket (with its associated life-support system) would need to weigh 100,000 kgm, then the mass of nuclear fuel consumed on the two-way journey would be about 36,000 kgm. No allowance has been made for the weight of the auxiliary equipment associated with the propulsion system. The general conclusion would seem to be that the technical problems of a 10-year round-trip to Alpha Centauri are enormous but not utterly outrageous. This star is, however, merely our next-door neighbour in the galaxy, at a distance of 1·3 parsecs. With the diameter of our galaxy at 25 *thousand* parsecs, the prospects of extensive visits seem slender indeed.

Are we however taking too unimaginative a view of the problem, by assuming the present-day form of propulsion? The arguments given above, concerning the energy required from the Centaurian journey are in fact general and do not depend on the form of propulsion. We have, however, tacitly assumed that all the nuclear fuel would need to be carried for the journey. Is there any alternative—e.g. could we "simply" collect the radiant energy from all the stars and, with suitable conversion, use this to propel the rocket? We think of the possibility of the laser here—if we can pump the laser with the energy collected from the stars (which streams in from all directions) and then operate the laser to give a beam in one direction only (an opaque mirror at one end of the cavity) then by virtue of the fact that a light beam carries momentum, there would be a reaction on the mounting. This may sound fanciful in concept. When the idea is exposed to a detailed analysis it does indeed prove to be quite impractical. The rate of collection of energy by such a process with a telescope system of human scale is many orders of magnitude too small for space journeys to be effected by this means at sensible rates.

It thus appears that, although the arrival of the laser may well facilitate the problems of communication and information transfer between spacecraft engaged in exploring the minute part of space accessible to us, there is no indication that the laser changes the scene so far as travelling range is concerned. Space is too big, too long-lived for beings with so transient an existence to be able to interact with more than the very closest part of his environment.

Military implications of the laser

There would appear to be two general areas in which the laser could influence future military developments. It is clear that its use will play a significant part in the development of conventional weapons. The scope for improved communication and the application of the laser to range-finding are two fairly obvious examples of the role which the laser can play. In view of the high power and energy capability, the question of its use as a direct weapon arises. It is certainly true that even the powerful laser of the present day is capable of producing lethal effects on human beings at moderate ranges. In a sense this is irrelevant. If the laser equipment required to kill is the size of a small cottage, it may not offer any great advantage over more conventional methods (such as the rifle). Even allowing for considerable further development, it does not at present appear that the laser will have any dramatic influence on conventional warfare.

The situation in respect of nuclear warfare is decisively different. It is perfectly possible to produce conditions, at the focus of a high-energy laser beam, such as are required to initiate a fusion reaction. Hitherto, the only method for producing the extremely high temperature which is needed for hydrogen fusion is that involving the explosion of a fission device, such as a uranium or plutonium bomb. Now the production of fission devices requires a highly-developed technology, operated on a substantial scale. It is for this reason that the manufacture of these weapons has for the most part been confined to the larger world powers. The step from the fission device to the fusion one is, however, a relatively simple one, requiring only moderate resources. Thus the emergence of a device which may lead to the chance of by-passing the fission bomb as a prerequisite for the hydrogen bomb could have a profound effect on the whole global power situation. For if the high-power laser can eventually be used to initiate fusion, it will be trivially easy for almost any national power to equip itself with hydrogen weapons. The technology required for the production of high-power lasers is entirely trivial compared with that needed for fission devices. It is a matter for speculation just how the international situation would develop if this became a reality.

Communication

If one examines the potentialities of the laser for the transmission of information, one may conclude that we are, even in the twentieth century, living in a state of incredible isolation. Whilst it is undoubtedly true that we have at our disposal truly immense amounts of information—in books, museums, periodicals—the time involved in our locating and then gaining access to such information can be very long. In addition, the sheer volume of available material is increasing now at an alarming rate. That the increase must eventually slow down is beyond doubt. If the law which describes the rate of increase of the weight of the journal "Physical Review" were to continue until the end of this century, the volume for the year 2000 would weigh more than the Earth. Ignoring the value judgment on whether the information which is being so assiduously stored is worth harvesting, the need clearly arises for methods of access to such information which differ radically from those used at present. In this area, the laser has much to offer and is almost certain to form a standard part of the information-handling and retrieval system of the future.

To deal first with the storage of information, we can see an immediate way in which the density of stored information can be increased, using laser technology, by an enormous factor over that represented by the printed page. A simple, direct method would be to form a hologram of the required page and to create a reconstruction when required by illuminating the hologram with a laser beam. Even with present-day recording materials (e.g. photographic plates) sufficient information to reconstruct a large page can be stored in a hologram less than one millimetre in diameter, where only two-dimensional storage is employed. If a thick emulsion is used, a very large number of pages could be stored in this way. This however is a very crude beginning to the solution of the storage and retrieval problem. It would require that the reader be in the neighbourhood of the recorded material. By the use, however, of television-type techniques, the reconstructed page image could easily be transmitted from a central (hologram) library to a receiver which may well be very far away. When we consider a system of this kind, however, it becomes clear that there is no need to store the information in the form envisaged, if more convenient ways exist, since all that is needed is a suitably reconstructed picture at the receiving end. In normal television techniques, the picture is transmitted as a series of pulses, and our information could well be stored in a form which allows the signal to be read off in this way. Thus we could envisage a series of dots imprinted on a suitable medium which are scanned by a laser beam. A detector placed behind the array of dots could then produce the desired electrical pulses. With the development of materials which can be coloured by exposure to a light beam, the information could be written by a laser. Reference has already been made to the *photochromics* which can be coloured by exposure to light of one colour and bleached by radiation of a different wavelength. These thus offer the possibility of an updatable information store, which can be revised as necessary.

The devices needed to store and retrieve information on a scale large compared with that represented by the British Museum Library are likely to be complex, so that only a small number of such central "libraries" would be provided. (At least two—in case one burned down!) The problem of access to and distribution of the information in such stores entails the provision of a set of information channels of considerable capacity. In this part of the system, the laser would be able, by virtue of its high frequency and its coherence, to provide all the capacity needed. The present problems which restrict the scope of laser communication in this form can be expected to be overcome in the not too distant future. A likely development in this direction is that of glass fibres, which—when the present problems of high loss are solved—will enable modulated laser beams to be carried in much the way that microwave signals are now distributed by cable.

There appears to be no reason why a laser-based system should not ultimately provide for all the required forms of communication on a domestic scale. A single fibre would be able to carry what is now received by radio and television, would handle telephone calls and would provide a link to the library, in which "books" are housed in the form of (probably digitally) stored information on crystals or magnetic devices. A dial or push-button call system, operated from the home, would enable the appropriate material to be selected, scanned, fed via the fibre to one's lounge where it would appear on a television-type screen. At a later stage, the information would be reconstructed holographically at the receiver, with the help of three lasers— red, green and blue—and would provide a three-dimensional colour reproduction of the material being studied.

Most of the above is within range of the technology which will be available by the early 1970s. The provision of live 3-D colour television on a domestic scale is somewhat more remote although there are no serious difficulties of principle. The pace with which this development occurs is likely to be determined by the rate of progress of research into the new materials which will be needed.

The issue which has already been raised in connection with the storage of personal information on present-day computers— that of personal privacy—will clearly become more and more important as the capacity for storing and handling information increases.

Biological/medical developments

The feasibility offered by the laser of producing highly localised spots of light has already indicated its use as a means of studying biological cells. In the region surrounding the nucleus of a cell, there are many minute systems, distributed throughout the cytoplasm, many of whose functions are not yet clear. Laser beams may be focused to points of size comparable with these cell sub-systems which may therefore be selectively destroyed.

Study of the form of the subsequent development of the cell thus enables the role of the treated sub-systems to be discerned. The next step may well be that of being able to determine the form of cell development by suitable treatment with laser beams. An allied possibility, under current discussion and for which there already exists some evidence, is that of influencing chemical reactions by the use of lasers, through the high field produced. The above two effects combine to suggest that genetic engineering on a molecular scale may become an eventual reality. As with the fruits of so many fields of human endeavour, a result of this type could be used in either a beneficial or a destructive mode. It would, for example, herald the possibility of eliminating hereditary congenital defects and of controlling diseases or deformity. The abuses to which a power of this magnitude could be put are too obvious to mention. It is perhaps fortunate that, even allowing for the very rapid pace of technological development which we are now witnessing, this situation is unlikely to arise for, at the very least, several decades. We have time to study the problems to which such developments give rise. In some respects, these represent perhaps the most far-reaching and difficult possible impacts of the laser on the future of civilisation. It is to be hoped that we are ready to deal with the situation when it arises.

Further reading

Andrade, E. N. da C., Silva, J. L., and Lochak, G. *Quanta*. New York: McGraw-Hill, 1969.

Brotherton, Manfred *Masers and Lasers*. New York: McGraw-Hill, 1964. Introduction by Charles H. Townes.

Heavens, O. S. *Optical Masers*. New York: Wiley, 1964.

Schawlow, Arthur L., ed., *Lasers and Light, Readings from Scientific American*. San Francisco: Freeman, 1969. See in particular "Optical Masers" and "Advances in Optical Masers" by Arthur L. Schawlow.

Spruch, G. Marmor, "The Laser's Grandfather", *Saturday Review*, March 4, 1967.

van Heel, A. C. S., and Velzel, C. H. F., *What is Light?* New York: McGraw-Hill, 1968.

Index